HEALING CRYSTALS

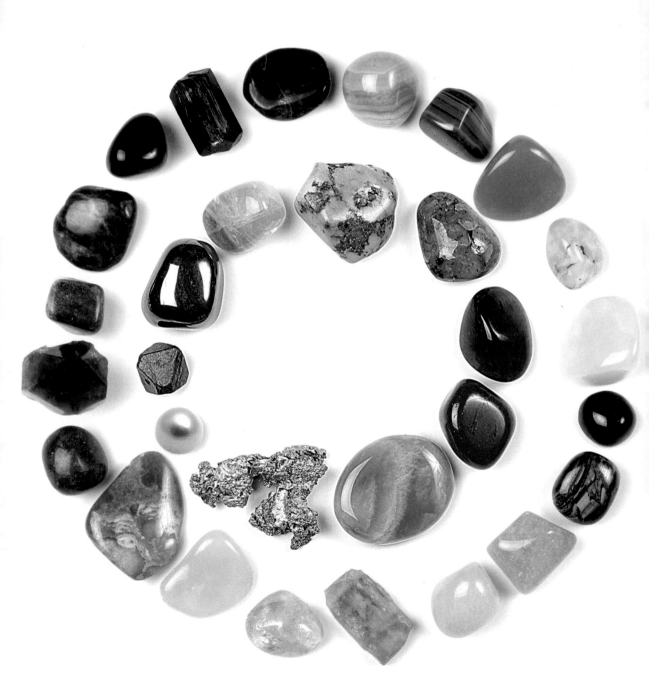

HEALING CRYSTALS

The Perfect Guide to Healing Your Heart, Mind, Body, and Soul with the Power of Crystals

Catherine Mayet &
Nathaëlh Remy

Skyhorse Publishing

CAUTION

People often talk about 'therapeutic' crystals, but the term is not used here in its strictly medical sense. Just as a piece of music or a book can have a healing effect, so too can crystals. Note that the applications suggested in this book should not be used to replace current medical treatment.

First Skyhorse Publishing Edition 2019

Text copyright © Catherine Mayet and Nathaëlh Remy/Leduc.s Éditions 2017
This edition copyright © Welbeck Non-Fiction Limited,
part of Welbeck Publishing Group Limited 2020

Skyhorse Publishing books may be purchased in bulk at special discounts for sales promotion, corporate gifts, fund-raising, or educational purposes. Special editions can also be created to specifications. For details, contact the Special Sales Department, Skyhorse Publishing, 307 West 36th Street, 11th Floor, New York, NY 10018 or info@skyhorsepublishing.com.

Skyhorse® and Skyhorse Publishing® are registered trademarks of Skyhorse Publishing, Inc.®, a Delaware corporation.

Visit our website at www.skyhorsepublishing.com.

10 9 8 7 6

Cover design by Fogdog Creative
ISBN: 978-1-63158-431-2
eISBN: 978-1-63158-440-4

Printed in China

First published in France in 2017 by Leduc.s Éditions as
Le Grand Guide des Pierres de Soin au Féminin

CONTENTS

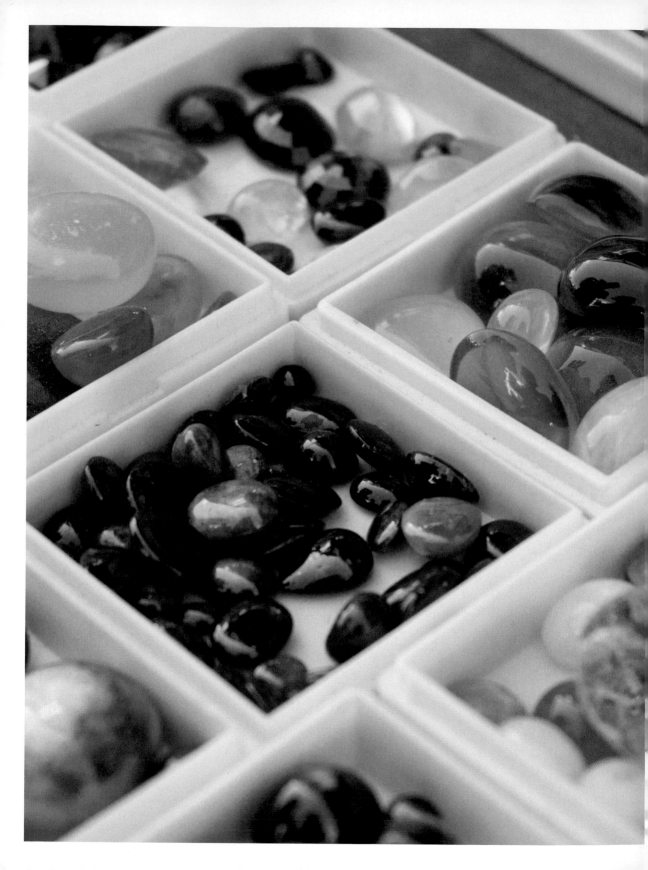

Welcome to the world of crystals

When you enter the crystal universe you discover a fascinating new world that brings joy and personal fulfilment. As female practitioners of lithotherapy, or crystal healing, we felt it was important to write a book for women who love crystals and want to work with them. These stones have a gentle power that can be used in myriad everyday ways to enhance femininity and well-being throughout the four stages of life – childhood, adolescence, adult life and motherhood, and later life. Using and handling these stones encourages happy emotions, and their effects can also boost intuition and enhance personal development.

As a general rule, several healing crystals are recommended and it is exciting to try them one by one or together to discover which work best with which season, with which state of mind or to achieve the healing effect desired. There are also crystals that are best held in the hand to enrich meditation or contemplation.

We suggest that you use a special notebook to jot down your experiences with different crystals. Observing and making a note of their effects on your general or emotional health will greatly help to raise your awareness and enable you to interpret the messages that the crystals are sending you.

Crystals & chakras: a story about colours

We should briefly touch on the concept of 'chakras' as they are related to crystals. The term 'chakra' comes from the ancient Sanskrit and means 'wheel' or 'disc'. According to Indian tradition, the chakras are the seven flowers or energy points of the human body. Each has a front and rear-facing side. Located the length of the vertebral column, the chakras are subtly linked to endocrine glands, which secrete hormones or other products into the blood, and are also a receptacle for emotions that we have experienced. Placing a crystal on its related chakra rebalances energy flow.

Each chakra corresponds to a musical note or a colour. Certain practitioners of magnet therapy and so-called clairvoyant healers describe them as funnels or types of vortices that suck in and emit energy. The renowned American scientist and healer Barbara Ann Brennan outlined their roles and functions very precisely in her book *Hands of Light*. Numerous other authors have written about chakras, but in our short account we have chosen to draw on her expertise.

A disorder or a simple malfunction in one organ inevitably creates an imbalance in its related chakra. This imbalance may be due to a psychological or emotional upset or to a failure to recognize some fundamental need. The crystal, via its colour, is the link to the chakra that bears the same colour. It is believed that the energy forces of a crystal resonate with its corresponding chakras, thus redressing the imbalance.

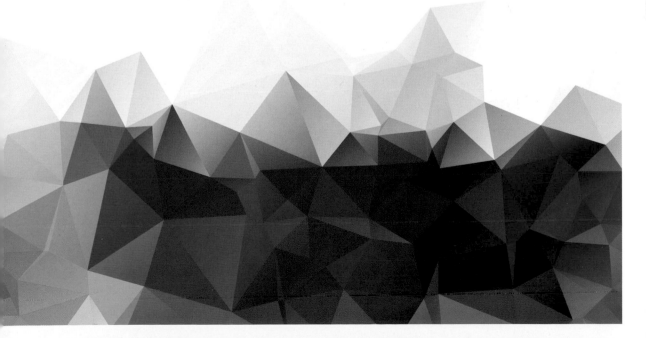

The chakras

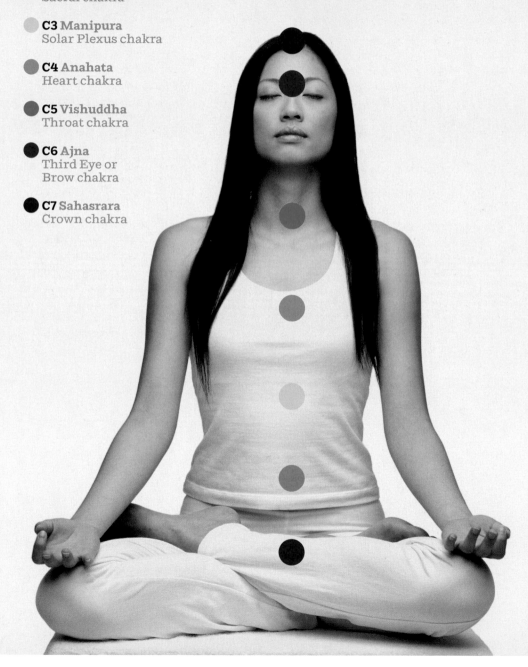

- ● **C1 Muladhara**
  Root or Base chakra
- ● **C2 Svadhisthana**
  Sacral chakra
- ● **C3 Manipura**
  Solar Plexus chakra
- ● **C4 Anahata**
  Heart chakra
- ● **C5 Vishuddha**
  Throat chakra
- ● **C6 Ajna**
  Third Eye or
  Brow chakra
- ● **C7 Sahasrara**
  Crown chakra

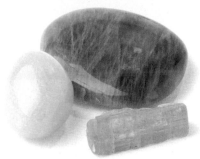

C1 Muladhara
Root or Base chakra

In the human body, the first chakra is located between the rectum and the perineum. It is linked to the kidneys and the adrenal glands, and also to the rectum and anus. Its associated colours are purple, red, brown and black. If problems occur in any of the zones related to this chakra, harmony can be restored by using a stone of the same hue as the chakra's associated colours.

The Root chakra is linked to survival, the desire to live in our physical reality. It gives us the ability to assert ourselves and provides a base and the stability to implement our plans. The crystals associated with this chakra enable us to achieve goals and anchor us in the material world. They encourage us to be more practical, more realistic and to keep our feet firmly on the ground.

The related crystals include:
red crystals: Red Garnet, Red Jasper, Ruby
brown crystals: Magnetite, Hematite
black crystals: Black Obsidian,
Black Tourmaline

C2 Svadhisthana
Sacral chakra

This chakra is located on the stomach, at about three finger widths below the navel. This is at the point called Hara, a Japanese term, which is considered the centre of vital energy. The endocrine (hormone-producing) glands involved here are the genital organs – for women, the ovaries, the Fallopian tubes, the uterus and the vagina. The colour associated with this chakra is orange. The Sacral chakra is connected with the reproductive system and also sexuality (giving pleasure and receiving it).

It plays an important role in the mother–child relationship. This centre of vital energy also helps to develop the inner creativity that all women possess. You just need to wear or carry one or more of its related crystals.

The related crystals are:
orange crystals: Imperial Topaz, Orange Calcite, Copper, Orange Moonstone

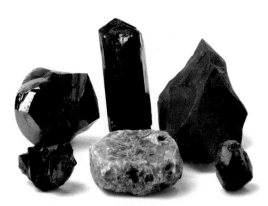

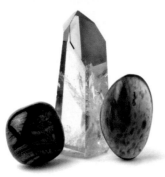

C3 Manipura
Solar Plexus chakra

This energy point radiates its power in the zone of the diaphragm. Its related endocrine gland is the pancreas. The stomach, liver, gall bladder and spleen are also linked with this chakra. Its associated colour is yellow. The Solar Plexus chakra is also involved with our connection to the Universe.

The related crystals are:
yellow crystals: Amber, Citrine, Imperial Topaz, Tiger's Eye

C4 Anahata
Heart chakra

This chakra covers the heart zone. It is the heart that gives rise to the feelings and emotions we experience towards family members, friends, professional colleagues, and all those we encounter, as well as towards the creatures that live on Earth. The Heart chakra's colours are green and pink. Some traditions also add gold. Healing via this chakra brings an awareness that love can transcend negative feelings.

The related crystals are:
green crystals: Chrysoprase, Chinese Green Jade, Emerald, Malachite, Green Aventurine, green Fluorite, Chinese green Turquoise
pink crystals: Rose Quartz, Rhodochrosite, Morganite, Ruby, pink Lepidolite

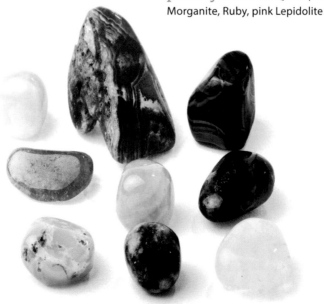

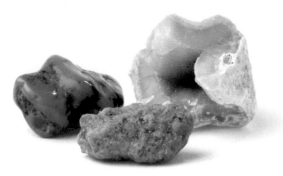

C5 Vishuddha
Throat chakra

This point is concerned with the throat and the associated endocrine gland is the thyroid. Other related areas are the respiratory system, the nose, the trachea, the bronchial tubes and the lungs. This chakra also affects speech and hearing. Associated colours cover the full range of light blues.

The related crystals include:
light blue crystals: Blue Chalcedony, Turquoise, blue Fluorite, Sapphire.

C6 Ajma
Third Eye or Brow chakra

The pituitary is the endocrine gland involved here. The brain, eyes and ears are all linked to the Third Eye chakra. This energy point is concerned with ideas and the ability to visualize. Its related colour is indigo but also a range of dark blue shades, sometimes with a starry shimmer if the chosen crystals have mica or pyrite inclusions.

The related crystals are:
dark blue crystals: Lapis Lazuli, blue Sapphire

C7 Sahasrara
Crown chakra

This chakra is situated at the crown of the head. Here the associated endocrine gland is the pineal gland. This chakra is linked to our spirituality and the way each of us perceive it. It allows us to experience spiritual moments. Its colour is purple, white or gold.

The related crystals are:
purple crystals: Amethyst, purple Fluorite, Lilac Lepidolite
golden crystals: Imperial Topaz, Citrine
white crystal: Freshwater Pearl

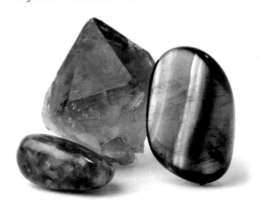

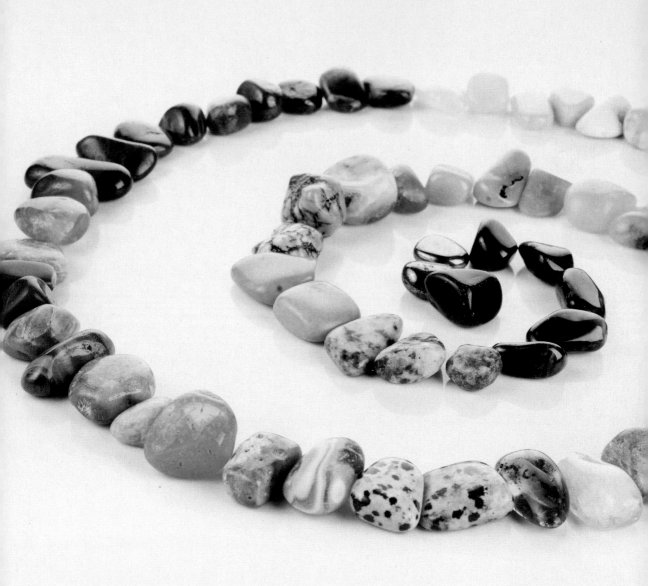

Basic principles

Before you discover which crystals attract you and meet your needs,
you must learn how to use them. Their effects on the body,
mind, soul and emotions will differ from person to person.
Pick and choose from the 30 crystals suggested here.

*This book features 20 essential crystals and
10 'bonus' crystals which work
in harmony with them.*

Healing crystals: 20 questions & answers

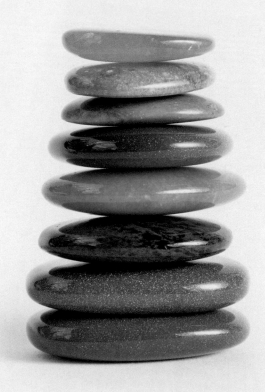

1 What is a healing crystal?

A therapeutic or healing crystal is a mineral which, depending on its properties, produces a beneficial effect. The healing qualities of the crystals featured here have been recognized since ancient times and acknowledged by certain visionaries such as, in the Middle Ages, the German saint Hildegard of Bingen. Since then, their properties have been further studied and evaluated as professional lithotherapists have recorded their own experiences and reactions. The beneficial effects of crystals can be emotional, invigorating or spiritual, which is why crystals are described as 'therapeutic'. In the event of illness, healing crystals can be a helpful addition to conventional medical treatment but should not be used as a substitute.

2 Where do these crystals come from?

The crystals are extracted from deposits that occur naturally throughout the world. Crystallized minerals differ in form according to the composition and temperature of the ground in which they were formed.

3 How do they transmit their powers?

There are several different hypotheses. Everything that exists on Earth, such as sound, light or colour, vibrates to a particular wavelength. Crystals resonate as a result of their colour, structure, the trace elements present during the original crystallization process, and the sum of their experiences since their formation. Crystals are also composed of minerals that humans need to replenish the body's mineral content. It is believed that a subtle transmission of power from the crystals will redress any mineral deficiencies in the body. The process occurs via skin contact with the crystal and also across electromagnetic fields. The vibrational resonance between a crystal and an individual facilitates imperceptible exchanges of information.

Meeting clients in the mineral store where we worked taught us some interesting and surprising things. For instance, we noticed that children aged under seven often experienced the power of crystals quite naturally. Some highly sensitive and receptive people retain that ability to communicate with the mineral world as they get older. However, most people say they feel nothing, most probably because they are not sufficiently capable of listening to their bodies. Wanting and deciding to hone this sense makes individuals aware of their own responsiveness, developing their capacity to communicate with crystals. It also helps people become less judgemental towards themselves and towards those who lack this responsiveness. In this way emotional or energy imbalances can be resolved. This is why we generally suggest using crystals directly on your skin to enhance and feel their effects, and to encourage the transfer of their mineral power.

4 Have the healing powers of crystals been scientifically proven?

As far as we know, the healing powers of crystals have not yet been scientifically confirmed. They are, we believe, subjective and therefore difficult to measure in this way. Can anyone actually assess and quantify a beneficial effect? Can it ever be the same for everyone?

5 How do they differ from hot stones?

Author's note

Nathaëlh I myself have used hot stones in thalassotherapy to give dedicated healing massages, working with a doctor at the treatment centre. The stones are volcanic and highly heat-resistant. The massage always ended by gently removing the hot stones and placing healing crystals such as donuts of Orange Calcite, Chinese Green Jade, Blue Chalcedony and Lapis Lazuli on the chakra points for several minutes. Before being put back into their heated tank, the volcanic stones were laid on a bed of salt for a time, then rinsed with spring water.

6 How are crystals linked to areas such as astrology or magnetism?

In astrology, crystals are defined in terms of the four elements – air, earth, water and fire – within which the 12 astrological signs are grouped. Practitioners of magnet therapy, or 'magnetizers', transfer healing energy to the client and will often themselves use crystals to reduce and to boost energy levels. Lithotherapists work with crystals, placing them on the client during a treatment session.

7 What different types of crystal are there?

Crystals are chosen for their beauty and their rarity value. Usually, they are carefully removed from rock and never suffer any kind of mishandling (other stones may be extracted using dynamite). Their weight can vary from tens of grammes to hundreds of kilos for Amethysts or huge blocks of Rock Crystal. They can be admired in museum displays, at mineral fairs and in stores that sell minerals or gems for export. The largest mineral fair in the world is the Tucson Gem, Mineral & Fossil Showcase that takes place annually in winter at more than 40 venues in Tucson, Arizona.

Mineral specialists from throughout the world can be found there. In France, the Mineral and Gem International Show is held each June in a pretty Alsace village called Sainte Marie-aux-Mines.

Semi-precious or precious stones, such as Diamonds, Rubies, Sapphires or Emeralds, are sold in jewellery shops. These gems are highly prized for their beauty, rarity, purity and quality. They will be cut and ground into forms that can be used in jewellery. Their weight is minuscule and is measured in carats (1 carat = 200 mg or 0.2 g). Set decoratively in jewellery as conspicuous symbols of power or wealth, these stones are offered as tokens of love and fidelity on occasions such as an engagement or wedding. However, semi-precious stones such as Amethyst, Turquoise, Jade, Rose Quartz and Moonstone are being used increasingly in jewellery workshops.

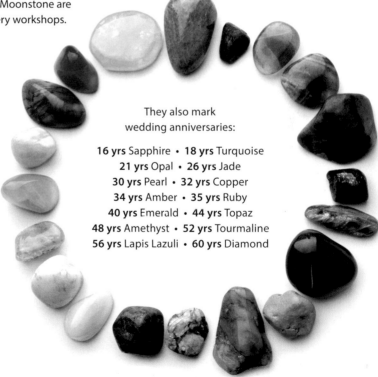

Jewellery set with semi-precious stones, that is all crystals except the precious stones, tends to be less expensive.

The crystals featured in this book are either raw or 'tumbled' (polished) and are smooth to the touch. Prices vary according to the size, quality and rarity of the particular crystal but are generally affordable.

They also mark
wedding anniversaries:

16 yrs Sapphire • **18 yrs** Turquoise
21 yrs Opal • **26 yrs** Jade
30 yrs Pearl • **32 yrs** Copper
34 yrs Amber • **35 yrs** Ruby
40 yrs Emerald • **44 yrs** Topaz
48 yrs Amethyst • **52 yrs** Tourmaline
56 yrs Lapis Lazuli • **60 yrs** Diamond

8 Are crystals beneficial in all their forms, whether on necklaces, bracelets or as part of other jewellery?

Whatever form it takes, the crystal's energy remains present. Nighttime encourages absorption of its healing powers, as the body and mind are at rest. You can, for instance, place the crystal under your pillow.

A necklace will be a little more expensive depending on its length and the number and quality of the stones. Different styles are suggested to suit individual preferences. It is always best to choose something which you find attractive.

A pendant is more unobtrusive. It can be worn alone on a chain or with other stones, according to taste and the desired effect.

A donut is a flat, round stone with a central hole, a shape that enables it to emit power in a wave effect, which accelerates its action on the chakras, especially during meditation. It can be easily laid or fixed in place on your skin at a precise point to achieve a more targeted effect. If you do this, choose a smaller stone that will be easier to use in this way. You will find them in lots of different diameters. Larger ones can be threaded with cotton or leather and worn round the neck.

Bracelets can be easily worn at any time around the wrist or ankle (see page 75, 'Making an anklet'), as can earrings.

A flat, polished stone in pebble form can be carried in your pocket, slipped or sewn into your bra, attached to the body or to a baby's stomach.

All the forms above are polished stones, which have been tumbled in water in a rotating barrel to wear them down and make them as smooth as the pieces of glass you find on the beach that have been cast up by the sea. As they have no sharp edges and are soft to the touch, they are easy and pleasant to use.

Uncut, or raw, crystals have not undergone any process such as cutting or polishing, so can be quite coarse and rough-edged. Raw Black Obsidian, for instance, is as brittle and sharp as glass.

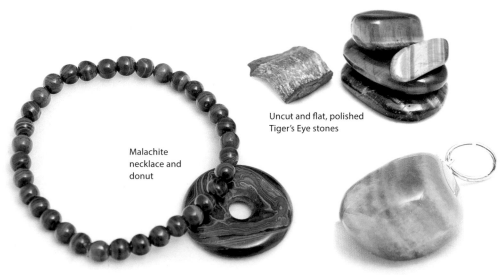

Uncut and flat, polished Tiger's Eye stones

Malachite necklace and donut

Orange Moonstone pendant

9 How should I choose a crystal?

Whether it is a spontaneous purchase or chosen for health reasons, you should let your heart guide you. A crystal must resonate with its user, as this creates a special bond. You have to follow your instincts and buy a crystal that pleases you. The amount of enjoyment and wonder people get from a crystal will vary according to each individual's personality.

Author's note

Nathaëlh One evening, a customer arrived with her little girl, who appeared to be about four years old. The mother walked around looking at various crystals, sometimes consulting the reference book she had with her. She called to her little girl to follow her, but the girl stayed at the front of the shop in front of the rows of uncut Rose Quartz crystals. She touched them several times while looking at her mother each time she was called. Seeing this, I went up to the little girl and, squatting down to her height, I asked her, 'Don't you want to join your mummy?' She replied timidly, 'No'. Smiling at her, I nodded towards the crystal and asked her, 'Is it telling you secrets?' Hesitating, the little girl said to me, 'Yes. It's stroking my hand and I feel it's like my soft, snuggly comforter.' I suggested she should stay there for a moment with the crystal.

10 How should I use a crystal?

You can hold the crystal in your hand, for instance, during a walk, or attach it to yourself with special sticky tape (available from pharmacies) that doesn't irritate the skin. You can also put it in your pocket or in your bra. Contemplation or simple meditation will help you to get in touch and commune with the crystal. For some people, this can be a very rich and surprising journey of self-discovery. Focusing on the crystal, you can experience it and absorb its light, colour and form.

If you forget to take it with you, you can visualize it or conjure it up in your imagination. Scientific studies now show that in this context the brain does not differentiate between imagination and reality.

At night, the mind is at rest but the body gets the chance to cleanse and regenerate itself. This is a good time to use a crystal, particularly over the long term. Whether you're doing this for yourself or a child, it's a good idea to place the crystal under the pillow or in the pillowcase so that it can have a subtle effect on the mind.

It is essential to clean the crystal regularly and re-energize it, following the instructions on page 24.

11 How can I 'train' and develop my awareness?

Whenever you come across a shop selling minerals, you should:

- **choose one or more crystals that attract you**
- **take the crystal and hold it in your hand, while listening to your inner awareness and focusing on your interaction with the crystal at that moment**

The power of a crystal can be felt in a number of different ways. It may, for instance, feel like a shiver or a tingle, or give you a sense of well-being or warmth or coolness. Emotions like joy and inner peace may also be experienced. The intensity of such sensations may vary. As you hold a crystal, these feelings may grow stronger or weaken but the stone will still be quietly working for your benefit.

At the start of your crystal 'apprenticeship', you may have only a faint awareness of a crystal's power. That is perfectly normal, as some people are not used to focusing on such feelings. Other very sensitive people require calm and silence in order to experience the power. Above all, it is essential to trust yourself and the response you feel, even if you cannot define or explain it. Your brain is on hold, but little by little your awareness is increasing.

With practice you will become more aware of a crystal's effect, which differs in intensity from person to person. We ask you to stay in touch with your feelings. You must be patient and listen to your body, as this process is gradual. Working with crystals is a long-term project but a very exciting one.

Working with crystal power: a step-by-step guide to boost well-being

1 Choose crystals whose weight, form, colour or other features appeal to your emotions and senses.

2 To keep warm, put on an extra sweater or wrap yourself up in a blanket. When you work with crystal energy, you may experience cold or heat.

3 Don't have your mobile phone near you or on you. Put it down some distance away so that it doesn't interfere with the energy field.

4 Remain clothed.

5 Rest on your bed, either lying on your back or sitting down, in whichever position is most comfortable.

6 Place your chosen crystals on your solar plexus.

7 Lay your hands over the stones without touching your body. Let them move gently, slowly or rapidly as you wish, for as long as you like. Your hands can trace different movements. Imagine, perhaps, the turning sails of a windmill. You could also gently move your hands as if you were caressing the energy of the stones that is radiating over your body.

8 At first your hands move in the space around the crystals, then towards the upper or lower part of the body. Work on the stomach if it feels knotted. If, however, you have a sore throat, draw the power of the crystals towards this area. To avoid tiring your hands, rest your elbows on the mattress.

9 To complete the session, you can rest there peacefully with the crystals in place or let yourself fall asleep if you are drowsy.

12 Can several crystals be used at once?

During consultations, we often use a selection of different crystals. Depending on the nature of the 'wounds' that need healing – the emotional problems or types of pain involved – people tend subconsciously to put up a protective screen. The self wears a psychological mask. Crystals can help people to discover or rediscover the nature of their inner soul. A good way of beginning your voyage of self-discovery is to start by concentrating on a single crystal and writing down your experiences in a personal notebook. When your interest flags, get to know a new crystal.

Crystals have a synergy and work together, complementing each other's power. For one person, a deep subconscious emotion may surface when using a particular crystal, while someone else will require a different crystal to access the same emotion. Each crystal that elicits an emotional response gives you a new healing stone and so your collection grows. A personal collection of healing crystals can vary from two to eight stones.

13 Are there any contraindications?

The crystals featured in this book can be used by everyone and pose no dangers. They are also easy to use. However, as mentioned, for anyone in poor health, crystal therapy can be helpful but is no substitute for conventional medical care.

14 Can crystals be used on a child?

Absolutely, and how to do so is fully explained in this book (see page 43). If a child is unwell, it is strongly advisable to consult a doctor and to continue using crystals if the child wants to do so.

15 What about pregnant or breastfeeding women?

Yes, they can use crystals, too. This subject is discussed in a later chapter (see page 104). Pregnant and breastfeeding women tend to be more emotionally aware at this point. Many women also become more intuitive. Surrounding yourself with beautiful crystals can be highly beneficial when coping with the discomforts of pregnancy, such as a weak bladder, and also at the start of breastfeeding when suffering from lack of sleep!

16 Can a crystal be lent to someone else?

A crystal will stay with its owner for a period or during certain times of life. It can be used by another person (after it has been cleaned), or perhaps offered as a present to someone who feels an affinity for a crystal that you can part with. Crystals are treasures of the Earth, so should be given to people who need them, especially if a person feels themselves drawn to a particular stone.

17 How do I clean, recharge and preserve my crystals?

CLEANING

Salt water: The best plan is to collect seawater from tidal marshes or from the beach, making sure it is pure. Alternatively, you can create a saline solution with demineralized water and natural sea salt or rock salt (salt crystals formed underground many millions of years ago). Use 30 g to 40 g (about 3 to 4 level teaspoons) of salt to one litre of demineralized water. A newly bought crystal should be left in this solution for 24 to 48 hours depending on its size, then rinsed and left to recharge.

Spring water: If you have the good fortune to live near a source of fresh spring water, such as one of the ancient 'lavoirs' (public wash-houses) that once existed on many European rivers, or a waterfall, or an unpolluted stream, make use of it, letting the water flow over your crystals. Afterwards, thank Nature for what she has done, then let the crystals recharge. Alternatively, you can buy a bottle of spring water.

Water with added clay: You can also put a few pieces of clay into a bowl or glass of water, let them dissolve and allow the crystals to soak overnight in this solution.

Fire: Crystals can be cleaned by lighting a candle and holding them over the flame for a few seconds.

Soil: If it gets a lot of use, a crystal may become discoloured or might crack. If this occurs, you must dig a small hole in the ground and bury the crystal for a while. When you do this, it is also important to thank the crystal for the experiences you have shared. The next year, you can unearth your crystal. You should expect to find it a little weathered. If it is still whole, but a little discoloured, it can be used again.

Dry clay: You can clean crystals by placing them on a bed of dry clay because it is a highly absorbent substance.

Scallop shell: The shell has a wave-like form, which gives it the power to clean a crystal, a crystal necklace, a donut stone or a bracelet. The crystal should be left in the shell for the night.

Cleaning soft, soluble crystals

Soft crystals whose particles might dissolve should not be cleaned with water, as they could disappear. Similarly, crystals that have some iron content, such as Hematite or raw Magnetite, should not be washed in water as they might corrode.

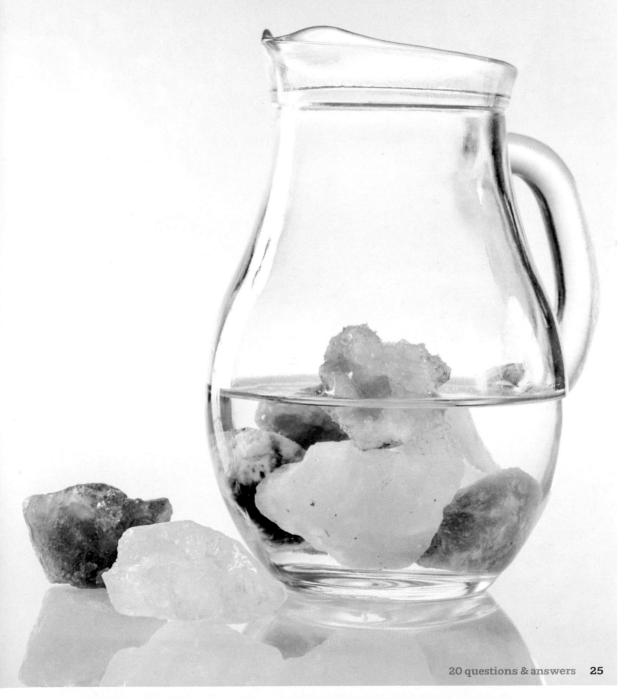

If cleaning with salt water, the best plan is to collect seawater from tidal marshes or from the beach, making sure it is pure.

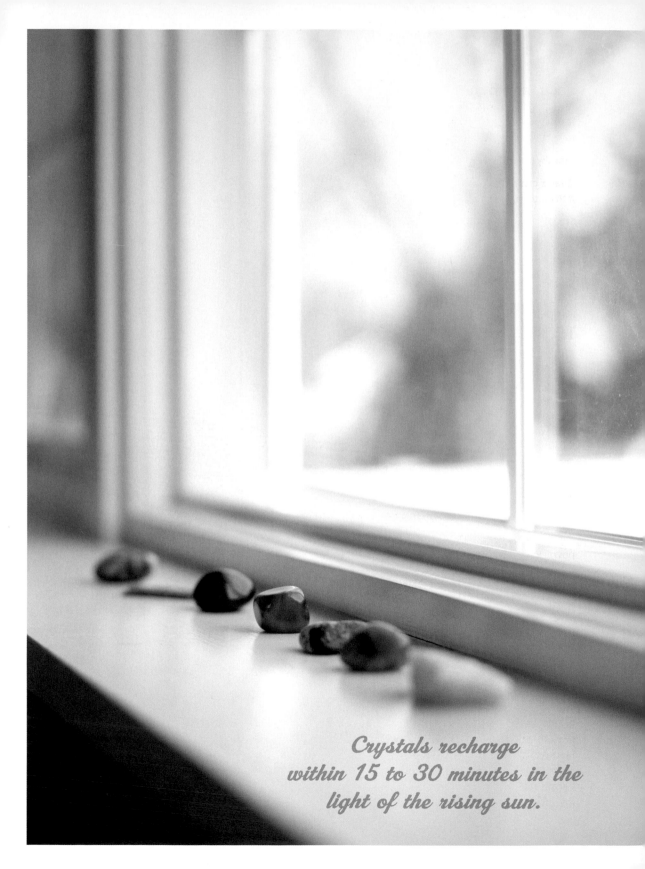

*Crystals recharge
within 15 to 30 minutes in the
light of the rising sun.*

RECHARGING

After you've cleaned the crystals, they will need to be recharged – that is, renewed and re-energized. When a crystal is carried or worn by someone, the intense force of energy transmitted can sap its power or it can become overloaded with unproductive energy.

Amethyst geode: Leave the crystal for at least half a day in the hollow of the geode.

Quartz crystal cluster: Lay the crystal down gently on the crystal cluster and leave it there to recharge for at least half a day.

Sun: When exposed to the light of the rising sun, crystals recharge within a maximum of 15 to 30 minutes.

Moon: In the light of a full moon, crystals also recharge within 15 to 30 minutes.

Storage: Crystals can be kept in an attractive box (see page 50) or in a fabric bag.

18 Where can I buy healing crystals?

Crystals can be very expensive in jewellery shops. The quality of the gem, its purity, the craftsmanship involved if it is a shaped, polished cabochon or teardrop, or if it is faceted, all add an extra cost, before you even consider the setting, which may be gold, silver or another precious metal. Such pieces are best offered as lovely gifts on special occasions.

The best place to buy a crystal for personal use is a shop that specializes in mineral specimens. It's advisable to go to several such stores and also to visit gem and mineral fairs or trade shows so that you can compare and contrast. Some internet sites also sell crystals, but take care when shopping online. Whether it's a present or for yourself, it's always preferable to see a crystal first-hand to assess the power of its attraction.

19 How do I judge the quality of a crystal?

It is best to buy your crystal in a reputable store. Some crystals are heated to alter their power and colour, which changes the nature of their vibrations. A heated Amethyst becomes an orange to yellow colour instead of its original purple and could therefore be sold as a Citrine. In that case, however, it would be rather opaque, whereas a natural Citrine is translucent. Coloured Howlite may also be passed off as Turquoise.

Some crystals are synthetic but these can usually be identified by their plastic texture and sometimes excessive brightness. It is rare to find them in specialized mineral shops and, if they are there, they will be labelled as such.

20 How much do they cost?

The crystals featured here are generally quite reasonably priced, at around £2–5/US $3–7. Because of their quality, some crystals, such as Lapis Lazuli, Turquoise, Rhodochrosite, Imperial Topaz, Garnet, Ruby and Sapphire, are rare and therefore cost a little more (at least £10/$13). If they are raw stones or tumbled, Rubies and Sapphires are not too expensive because they are opaque. Those used in jewellery are very expensive, because they are cut and translucent.

The power of crystals

Crystals have numerous powerful properties that we attribute to them as a result of our own experiences with the stones, our sensitivity to them and our personal narrative. Remember that their effects are felt by some people and not by others. These effects are subjective and cannot be scientifically reproduced.

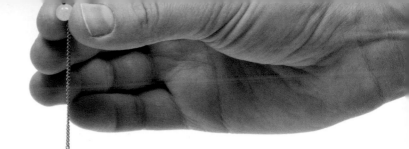

It is well worth considering what the late Dr Jacqueline Bousquet said in her book *Le réveil de la conscience* ('Awakening awareness'), mentioned earlier (see page 18). She explained that, beyond matter and their material form, minerals and metals were also made up of *vibrations-informations* – 'vibrational data'. She stressed the underlying concept of electromagnetic fields being the data medium.

The data that the crystals transmit via electromagnetic frequencies interacts with the chakras to balance the body's energy flow.

So what can crystal power do for us?

Effects on the mind: controlling emotions

On an emotional level, crystals can help us to change or manage difficult situations. They can fill a void or temper excessive or negative feelings, bringing them to the surface so we can decide to handle them in a positive way. They stimulate us to make positive changes and encourage personal development in each individual. Crystals strengthen our positive energy; like a sponge they absorb anything that disturbs our equilibrium, including negative emotions such as anger and jealousy. After use, however, it is essential to wash a crystal that carries one or more of these negative feelings so that it can recover its purity. Then it must be recharged to restore its original power. Intuitive people, such as lithotherapists, can sense negative energy. You can sometimes feel it in certain rooms or in houses where the atmosphere is oppressive.

For example, after an argument, an obsessive thought that could give rise to anger becomes lodged in the solar plexus. An Orange Calcite crystal will bring tranquillity and gentleness to this energy point, while you can add a Rose Quartz to heal the emotional wound, a Lapis Lazuli to calm the mind or a Sapphire to develop your capacity for understanding other people.

Effects on the body: treating physical disorders

A crystal rebalances energy flow. It dissolves blockages, and heals or strengthens whichever part of the body needs it.

It is like a crutch, a support whose touch is reassuring. It can also be an emotional prop for those who feel misunderstood or very alone. Whatever effect is required, whatever you are seeking and whichever crystals attract you at that moment, you can be sure that they will work together for your well-being.

Effects on the soul: the sacred touch

A crystal helps you to discover yourself so you can better understand your reactions or defence mechanisms that unconsciously come into play when your emotions are disturbed. The stone leads you to meditation and spirituality. Being with it, in silence, our state of consciousness changes. The crystal takes us beyond the known into a dimension that is altogether larger than our everyday world. It encourages an enhanced sense of awareness and self-knowledge that will be individual and specific to each person. Crystals empower their users to discover their individual spirituality, their divinity.

The 20 essential healing crystals

There are many different crystals, so here we are featuring the 20 crystals (with 10 'bonus' crystals to follow) that work best for female problems and disorders. This handy selection will give you all the information you need to start using your crystals to their full potential.

The crystals are numbered from 1 to 30. These numbers are used in subsequent chapters for easy reference.

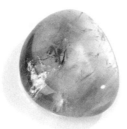

1 Amethyst

This Quartz crystal, which comes in varying shades of purple, calms anger, and soothes and banishes dark and sad thoughts. It relieves headaches and digestive problems that result from overeating. Amethyst will also help you to fall asleep and to cope with withdrawal symptoms. Note: A geode of this stone can help recharge other crystals.

2 Green Aventurine

This stone comes in varying shades of green and may also have pyrite or mica inclusions. It is gentle and comforting. It soothes problems of the heart and strengthens a couple's love. Green Aventurine will also help you cope with grief and will encourage you to make the best decision in a difficult situation.

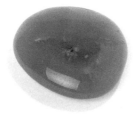

3 Blue Chalcedony

This is an Agate stone in varying shades of blue and may be mixed with or contain little ribbons of Agate or Milky Quartz. It allows you to express your thoughts, combating shyness. It reduces stress and frustration. It encourages sleep and will also drive away children's nightmares. It conveys serenity and its gentleness comforts the mind and soothes disturbed emotions.

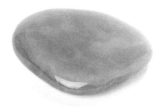

4 Orange Calcite

Ranging in colour from orange to yellow, this crystal immediately gives an impression of light. Its power can banish gloom, raise hopes and breathe joy into your life to support you when you feel down. It encourages balance on every level. It propels you towards self-confidence. It helps infants learn how to walk and convalescing patients to regain mobility. It also has a positive effect on digestion.

5 Chrysoprase

This apple-green to yellowish Chalcedony crystal encourages spark and drive. It is reassuring, helping you to stand back and accept change. It allows you to make decisions with your heart. It transmits a feeling of contentment that enables you to welcome new experiences. With this crystal you will find it easier to pamper yourself, take care of yourself and develop your femininity. It controls over-emotional feelings and alleviates the sadness resulting from a miscarriage. It calms pain in the womb or the ovaries, while encouraging ovulation. It clears the sinuses and balances stress.

6 Citrine

This yellow Quartz, whose luminosity varies according to its translucence, enhances concentration. It clears the mind, allowing you to take positive action. It reinforces creativity, good humour and joie de vivre. In relationships, it revitalizes the spirit of someone whose heart is tormented by jealousy. This crystal combats morning sickness in early pregnancy. In certain types of depression, it is the light at the end of the tunnel.

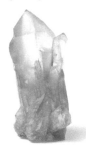
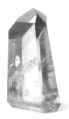

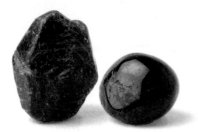

7 Red Garnet

This flaming red stone boosts blood circulation and relieves aching, tired legs. It helps you to implement projects and get things moving. It encourages you to listen to other people's views. It helps you develop creativity and courage. It warms you up and stimulates sexual desire.

8 Chinese Green Jade

This crystal, whose colour varies from light to deep green, encourages the development of wisdom and honesty. It tempers jealousy in envious people and removes a sense of guilt or injustice. It has a harmonizing effect and helps to ease temporary fatigue. Jade is also reassuring during childbirth. It is a real lucky charm!

9 Lapis Lazuli

This dark indigo-coloured stone, sometimes veined with Quartz and/or with pyrite or mica inclusions, looks like a starlit sky. Lapis Lazuli calms a troubled mind and helps you to fall asleep. It encourages intuition and listening to your inner self. It soothes insect stings and eyestrain caused by computer screen glare. It relaxes the chest after an asthma attack. The crystal also heals skin problems, helps combat withdrawal problems and alleviates headaches that are caused by worries or lack of sleep.

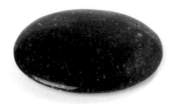

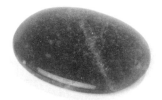

10 Lilac Lepidolite

This lilac and sometimes pinkish crystal, which is part of the mica family of stones, appears to be made up of tiny leaves laid one on top of the other. As a result, unpolished stones are quite fragile. This crystal brings joy and good humour. It reduces and relieves the symptoms of bipolar disorder. It calms obsessional thoughts, and is therefore helpful in combating withdrawal symptoms and the types of depression where the sufferer dwells on past events. It is reassuring for those who feel abandoned. Its lithium content has a beneficial effect on the nervous system, relieving shakiness and calming over-emotional feelings.

11 Malachite

Malachite comes in a wide range of greens, giving the crystal the appearance of a topographical map. The stone calms headaches caused by liver problems resulting from excessive alcohol intake or eating too many fatty or sugary foods. The crystal is helpful during childbirth and also reduces bruising by dispersing the collected blood.

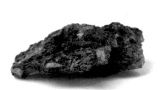

12 Morganite

This pink to light orange variety of Beryl may be opaque or translucent depending on the purity of its original crystallization. When confronting fear of the unknown, it is reassuring. It absorbs the shock of violent emotional upsets and relieves sadness, even when related to events long past. Morganite acts on the heart, encouraging acceptance, understanding and forgiveness. Its gentle vibrations fill the void when affection is lacking, bringing a sense of harmony and contentment.

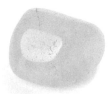

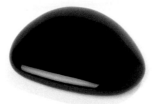

13 Black Obsidian

This shiny black crystal is as fragile as glass and will break easily if dropped or knocked. It has a grounding effect and brings clarity to our awareness, firmly dispelling illusions and fantasies. It relieves sadness and is a comfort during the grieving process. On the physical side, it combats muscle stiffness and cramping.

14 Tiger's Eye

This hazel-brown stone, which has a natural chatoyancy, or optical reflectance, can act like a mirror, deflecting whatever thoughts someone else has of us. It alleviates pain and regenerates tissue, encouraging wounds to heal. It gives you courage and enables you to work on plans and put them into action. It helps you reconnect with your inner self when a weakened emotional state of mind makes you feel as if you're living in a fog.

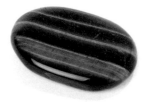

15 Rose Quartz

As its name suggests, this Quartz crystal has a gentle rose colour of varying intensity. It restores and strengthens relationships damaged by quarrelling. It controls excessively emotional feelings. This crystal soothes away doubt and calms the fear of being abandoned. It also encourages peaceful, restorative sleep.

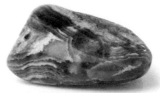

16 Rhodochrosite

Rhodochrosite builds emotional strength and, by tempering extreme feelings, helps to control anger. It has a restraining effect and encourages better communication. When excessive stress has an emotional cause, this crystal brings calm. The stone, which comes in varying pretty shades of rose pink, can relieve deep-rooted sorrows present and past. It controls the emotional fluctuations caused by female hormones. It brings resentments to the surface and helps overcome them by encouraging acceptance. Where there are conflict situations, it encourages a positive exchange of views and reduces tension. It also awakens a dormant libido.

17 Ruby

This crystal, which comes in shades of deep pink to red depending on how it was originally formed, helps to boost vitality. It is a powerful energizing force that also strengthens willpower. It supports determination, encouraging you to carry out and complete projects. It balances your mental state when emotions overwhelm you and pull you down. It restores your freedom to act and think clearly. It drives away tiredness and encourages healthy blood circulation.

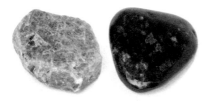

18 Sapphire

This gemstone, which comes in varying shades of bluish grey to blue, calms anxiety. It soothes hypersensitive reactions, encouraging a conciliatory response. It helps put matters into perspective.

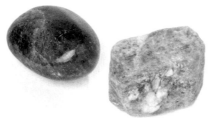

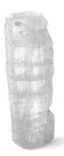

19 Imperial Topaz

This crystal's bright orange to yellowish colour and its translucence instil serenity. It also encourages self-awareness. It banishes morose feelings, replacing them with sparkling, contagious good humour. It teaches patience and heals emotional wounds. It brings tenderness to romantic relationships. It reassures those who feel lost and also soothes colic in babies.

20 Black Tourmaline

This brittle, linear black crystal may be veined with Milky Quartz or mica. It encourages you to feel anchored during meditation or relaxation sessions. It enhances awareness and tranquillity. Provided it is cleaned and recharged regularly, it protects against electromagnetic waves from electronic devices.

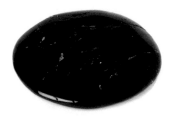

The 10 'bonus' crystals

Just as certain herbs or spices can enhance a recipe, these additional 'bonus' crystals can add something special to the 20 basic stones suggested. They extend the range of crystal healing possibilities and can be used at all stages of a woman's life.

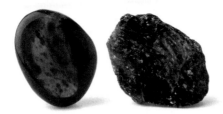

21 Amber

This stone is composed of organic tissue from fossilized conifers. Coloured yellow to brown and occasionally green, Amber can be carried or worn from early infancy to reduce the pain of teething and other mouth problems such as ulcers and inflamed gums. It appears that sucking a piece of Amber can also relieve throat problems and coughing bouts. In addition, this crystal helps treat disorders associated with older age.

22 Copper

This yellow-orange mineral is known for its ability to relieve pain. It invigorates the blood and strengthens morale. It also appears to have antibacterial properties. Copper helps to counter digestive disorders by acting on the liver and the gall bladder. It encourages skin regeneration as well.

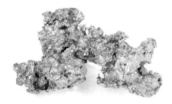

23 Emerald

This deep green Beryl gemstone can be veined with black. Emerald relieves tired eyes. It also has a remarkable ability to heal skin problems. It treats teenage acne and slows skin ageing. It sustains existing relationships and creates an awareness of the value of family bonds.

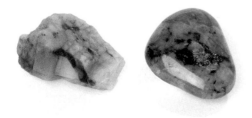

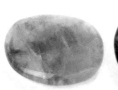

24 Fluorite

Depending on how it was originally formed, Fluorite may be plain, bi-coloured or multicoloured. Its fluoride content strengthens tooth enamel, improves bone density and keeps cartilage supple. Fluorite aids concentration during exams; for this purpose a blue stone is best. It also develops creative thinking. Yellow Fluorite is very helpful for gestational diabetes, the type that can develop during pregnancy. Green Fluorite clears emotional blocks and purple Fluorite unlocks the spirituality that every woman possesses.

25 Hematite

This metallic stone which has a high iron content stimulates the production of haemoglobin (red blood cells), especially during and after menstruation. It prevents tiredness at this time and regulates body temperature.

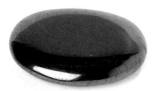

26 Red Jasper

This opaque stone, sometimes veined with black or white, connects us to the Earth. Red Jasper allows projects to take root so they can develop and come to fruition. It strengthens the survival instinct and is strongly recommended for deep depression, as it boosts morale. It encourages dynamic thinking and inspires courage.

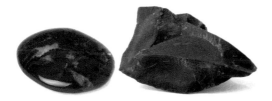

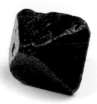

27 Magnetite

This metallic and naturally magnetic stone is a link to the core of the Eearth. This is why when you use it for meditation, Magnetite helps you to make wise decisions. It is recommended for relaxing cramped muscles. It helps you to centre yourself and resurface when a stream of brooding thoughts pulls you under.

28 Freshwater Pearl

A Freshwater Pearl is a natural gemstone, produced spontaneously by a freshwater pearl oyster. Its colour depends on the mollusc that forms it, so it may be white, orange or pink. It soothes nervous stomach pains and helps a woman to feel more attractive.

29 Orange Moonstone

This pearly orange and grey-white crystal regulates the menstrual cycle. It encourages fertility and comforts grief after a miscarriage or the death of a newborn.

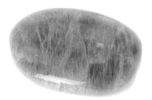

30 Turquoise

This porous stone, whether blue if from Arizona mines or green if from China, brings good luck. It protects against accidents, encourages good communication and combats shyness. It is also helpful for public speaking.

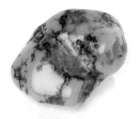

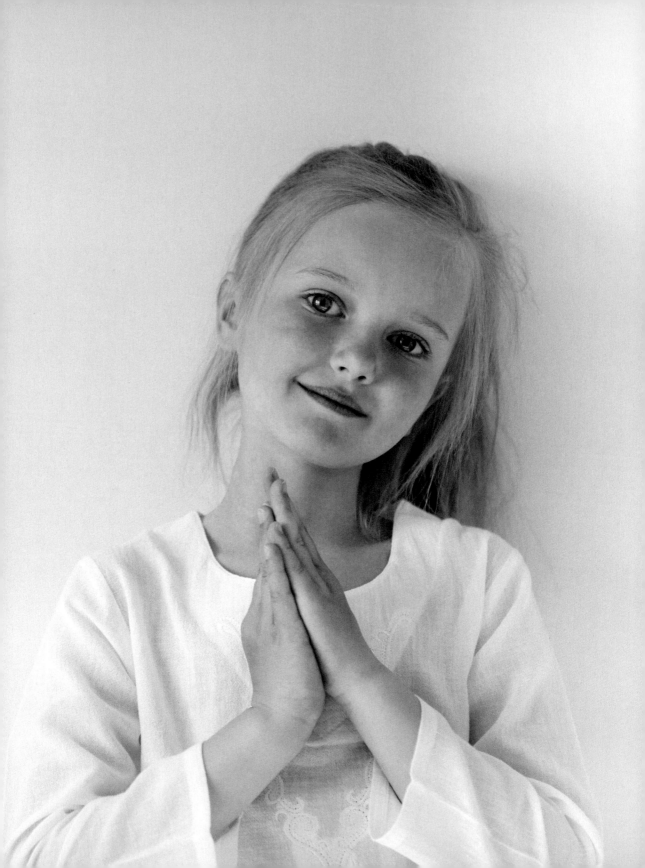

Healing crystals
for babies and little girls

From infancy and up to around the age of ten, a little girl will experience many different emotions that will cause her varying degrees of pain. A young child is guided only by her feelings, which can sometimes be quite overwhelming. Her ability to understand and reason is not developed enough to put them into perspective. For mothers, patience is key, at least until the child is more intellectually and emotionally mature.

Let's take a look at the crystals that can help to navigate through all of this!

Babies

As soon as a wonderful baby girl is born, she becomes an integral part of her mother's life. A mother has the joy of cuddling her and also breastfeeding, if she wishes to and can. At this age, an infant will encounter her first problems - weaning, digesting food, colic, adjusting to other carers, as well as teething, night fears and taking her first steps.

Digestive problems
When your child has colic

19 Imperial Topaz

21 Amber

22 Copper

4 Orange Calcite

Colic is a build-up of internal gas that creates discomfort and causes pain. It is often linked to milk intolerance or to dietary changes. A tumbled yellow or orange piece of *Imperial Topaz,* laid on the stomach in direct contact with the skin, can calm this disorder. The crystal can be held in place with a band. Green *Amber* will also prove very helpful, as will *Copper,* which calms digestive upsets. *Orange Calcite* stimulates the gastric juices so that the body can better absorb casein, the milk protein that often causes abdominal discomfort.

Separation anxiety
Leaving your child with a nanny or carer

10 Lilac Lepidolite

15 Rose Quartz

19 Imperial Topaz

1 Amethyst

9 Lapis Lazuli

The first – and greatest – fear of any baby is her mother's absence. If the mother has to be away for any length of time, the baby's most immediate concern is that she will never see her again. This feeling can develop into a sense of being abandoned. A piece of *Lilac Lepidolite* will calm distress and subconscious fears while also treating the nervous system. A piece of *Rose Quartz* slipped beneath her bedsheet can be useful for reassuring an infant. It is known that a child's fears can be unconsciously linked to the mother's fears, so a mother should use the same crystals as her baby but choose larger stones. She should take care of herself and explain the situation to her baby. *Imperial Topaz* is reassuring and counters any feeling of being abandoned. *Amethyst* is very gentle and helps the baby to accept a 'hardship' that is necessary for her personal development. *Lapis Lazuli* acts in a similar way, enhancing awareness.

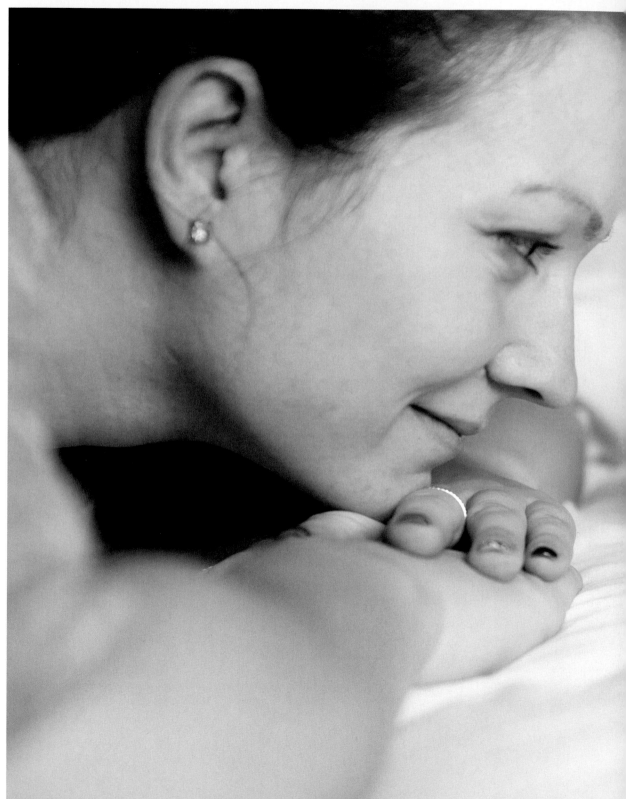

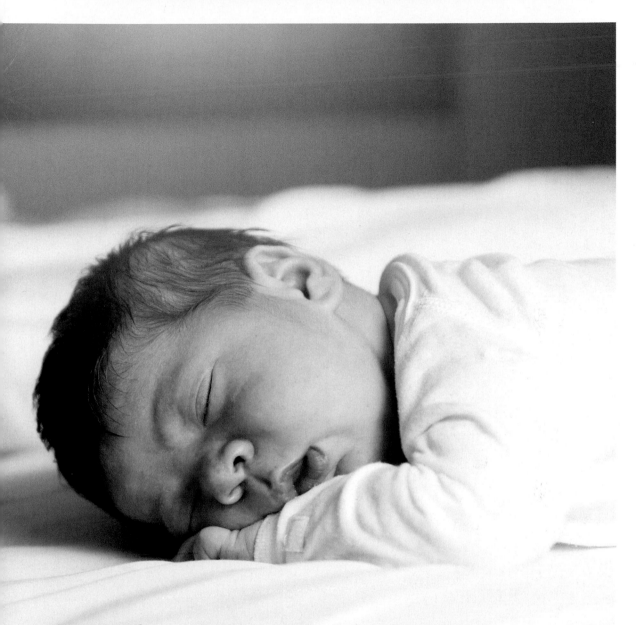

As soon as a wonderful baby girl is born, she becomes an integral part of her mother's life.

Weaning
When breastfeeding ends

1 Amethyst

9 Lapis Lazuli

10 Lilac Lepidolite

19 Imperial Topaz

Breast milk is both a physical and emotional food. The skin contact that occurs during breastfeeding offers both mother and child an intimate experience that binds them closely together. The transition from breast to bottle can be a difficult one. *Amethyst* helps to bridge the emotional gap that both may experience at this time. It is advisable for mother and daughter to wear a donut of amethyst or an amethyst necklace. *Lapis Lazuli* provides reassurance during weaning, subtly conveying the wisdom to accept that this step is an essential part of growing up. *Lilac Lepidolite* helps to calm anxious, crying infants, settling their mood and making them happy. *Imperial Topaz* combats feelings of abandonment and encourages independence and individuality.

Sleep problems
Night terrors and nightmares

15 Rose Quartz

2 Green Aventurine

3 Blue Chalcedony

19 Imperial Topaz

9 Lapis Lazuli

30 Turquoise

An infant can suffer significant fears and anxieties at bedtime. A large piece of raw *Rose Quartz* placed under the child's bed at head level will encourage peaceful sleep and will drive away night terrors. *Green Aventurine* relieves sadness, while *Blue Chalcedony* calms tearfulness. *Imperial Topaz* brings joy and comfort. Each of these crystals should be worn next to the skin on a necklace or pendant or secured under a stomach band. *Lapis Lazuli* gets rid of nightmares and should be slipped beneath the bedsheet of a baby, as should *Turquoise,* which combats sleep disturbances in young babies.

Teething
The first baby teeth

21 Amber

24 Fluorite

An *Amber* necklace will soothe a crying baby who is suffering teething pains. Such necklaces can be bought in specialist stores and online. A baby will instinctively suck her Amber necklace, so you should choose one that is long enough for her to do so or put the necklace beneath her bedsheet at night. As its name suggests, *Fluorite* contains traces of fluoride which strengthens tooth enamel. When all the milk teeth have fallen out, it is advisable to place a flat multicoloured piece of Fluorite beneath the child's bedsheet at night.

Learning to walk
First steps

14 Tiger's Eye

4 Orange Calcite

5 Chrysoprase

Time flies … and suddenly your baby is ready to walk. Moving from crawling on to two feet is an adventure. *Orange Calcite* helps her to take her first steps. It will give her the courage and confidence to make her first exploratory moves. When she's been walking for a short time while holding on to furniture or someone's hand, *Tiger's Eye* will give her the self-assurance to let go and move forward on her own. *Chrysoprase* will be useful now to encourage her sense of pride in growing up. These stones can be used in donut form or on a pendant.

Little girls

It is worth letting a little girl choose her own crystals. If she's given a free choice, the child will instinctively know which ones will be good for her. Later, under the influence of school, education and the media, she will sadly forget that she has these intuitive senses.

A casket of treasures from the Earth

When she joins other children at nursery and later primary school, a little girl will not be allowed to wear or carry a crystal. So then it will be best to put one or more of her chosen stones in a sachet or pouch tucked into her pillowcase or under her bedsheet. In this way, their healing power will work during her sleep. As a game, it is also fun to create a casket of 'Treasures from the Earth' and put all her prized crystals in it. The child can then pick out for herself whichever stone she wants to suit her needs or feelings at that moment. When she is old enough to use a pencil, she can also start recording her thoughts about the stones, scribbling and colouring in a notebook. Here is a suggested list of stones for her personal collection:

blue (Blue Chalcedony, Turquoise, Lapis Lazuli, Sapphire); **pink** (Rose Quartz, Rhodochrosite, Morganite, Ruby, Lilac Lepidolite); **green** (Green Aventurine, Chrysoprase, Emerald, Chinese Green Jade, Malachite); **yellow** (Amber, Citrine, Copper); **purple** (Amethyst, Lilac Lepidolite); **white** (Freshwater Pearl); **chestnut** (Tiger's Eye); **orange** (Orange Moonstone, Orange Calcite, Imperial Topaz); **black** (Black Tourmaline, Hematite, Magnetite, Black Obsidian); **red** (Ruby) and **multicoloured** (Fluorite).

Sadness
When the tears flow

4 Orange Calcite

6 Citrine

19 Imperial Topaz

Joy is innate and natural but also a fragile emotion in young girls, who can be extremely sensitive. Problems at school, rivalries and the fear of not having friends can be destabilizing and can make her afraid. If your child isn't playing as much or smiling as much as usual, her natural joy will need a boost, as joy banishes fear. *Orange Calcite* relieves sadness. *Imperial Topaz* brings joy. *Citrine* restores optimism and increases self-confidence. She can wear these crystals on a necklace, pendant or bracelet, or carry them in her pocket.

Jealousy
Breaking its grip

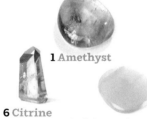

1 Amethyst

6 Citrine

8 Chinese Green Jade

23 Emerald

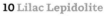

3 Blue Chalcedony

11 Malachite

9 Lapis Lazuli

10 Lilac Lepidolite

4 Orange Calcite

From time to time, a little girl can feel she is competing with her brothers and sisters, and may become afraid that she is not loved. As a result, she may choose to withdraw and cut herself off. There are several crystals that can help, whether worn on a necklace or pendant, or put in her pocket or under her pillow. *Citrine* and *Amethyst* will combat bouts of jealousy. *Chinese Green Jade* conveys wisdom and a sense of fairness. *Emerald* can complement the effects of Jade and is useful for forging harmonious relationships within the family circle. *Orange Calcite* will give the child the confidence she lacks and stop her wanting to play up. *Blue Chalcedony* will help her to express herself in a calm, controlled manner, while *Malachite* will relieve the frustration she feels about not understanding things. *Lilac Lepidolite* gets rid of the bad feelings caused by competitiveness and *Lapis Lazuli* helps to break emotional dependency.

Tantrums
Calming pent-up anger

1 Amethyst

19 Imperial Topaz

6 Citrine

4 Orange Calcite

16 Rhodochrosite

11 Malachite

26 Red Jasper

15 Rose Quartz

Tantrums occur for a number of different reasons. *Imperial Topaz* will calm a temperamental child. *Malachite* helps to control tantrums by making her aware of the cause of her anger. *Orange Calcite* will make her less emotional. *Citrine* enables a little girl to grow up and find her rightful place and discover the confidence she lacks. After a violent outburst, *Red Jasper* allows her to unwind. Because it opens the heart, *Rhodochrosite* resolves conflicts. *Rose Quartz* will comfort her if she feels unloved. *Amethyst* can turn around negative thoughts. These stones can be used as she wishes, on a necklace, in donut form, on a pendant, or as raw or tumbled stones, and can also be kept in her pocket or under her pillow.

Resentment
Stop that endless brooding

11 Malachite

5 Chrysoprase

2 Green Aventurine

Malachite helps to soothe the resentment and unresolved anger that a little girl may harbour. It helps her to let go and accept the situation. *Chrysoprase* allows her to put a past experience into perspective. *Green Aventurine* will help her to recognize and accept her own and the other person's anger. She can choose from these three crystals as she wishes or needs to, using them in donut form, on a pendant or a bracelet.

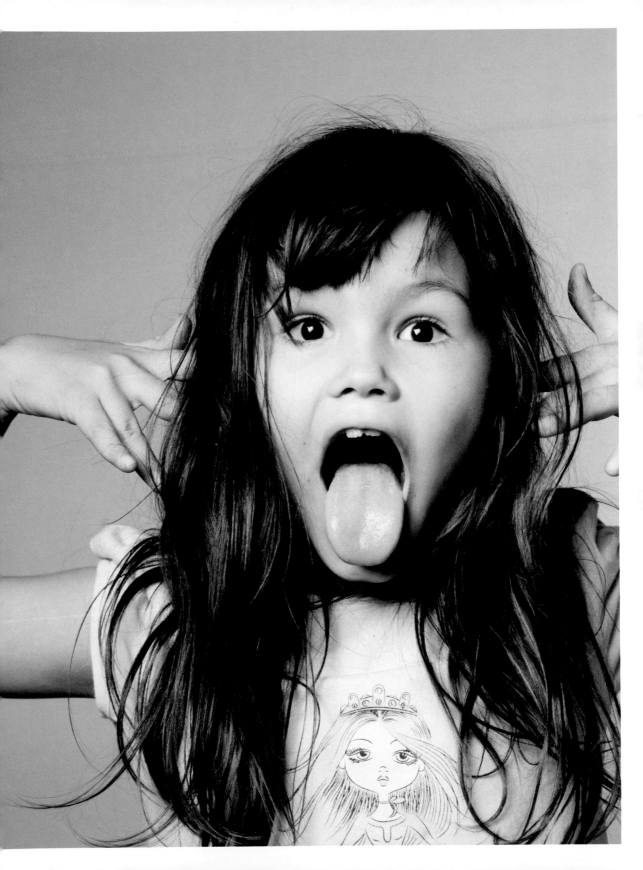

Childhood games

Brain specialists have discovered that laughing, playing and having fun are essential for a child to encourage the development of healthy neurons and a healthy brain. Guessing or hide-and-seek or other games with the crystals can be played in minutes and will reinforce the mother–daughter bond, and yield enormous present and future benefits.

Bad behaviour
I want this, I want that!

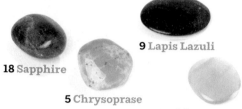

18 Sapphire

9 Lapis Lazuli

5 Chrysoprase

8 Chinese Green Jade

Lapis Lazuli together with *Chrysoprase* (on a pendant or in donut form) help a child to control her whims and do what she should. *Chinese Green Jade* helps her keep a sense of proportion. *Sapphire* will encourage her to speak gently rather than aggressively; this crystal can be worn on a necklace or pendant, or used in donut form.

Hypersensitivity
Emotional upsets, shock or traumatic events

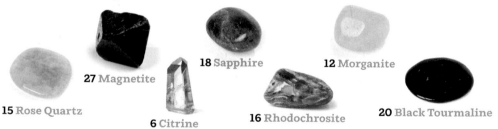

15 Rose Quartz

27 Magnetite

6 Citrine

18 Sapphire

16 Rhodochrosite

12 Morganite

20 Black Tourmaline

Children are not always gentle with each other and are often critical. Some take an unhealthy pleasure in putting down their friends. *Rose Quartz* can provide the love and tenderness that is lacking in such situations. *Magnetite* will help a child to remain anchored and stable. Certain life experiences or scenes of violence on television can have lasting effects on a child.

Sapphire, worn on a necklace or pendant, has a rebalancing effect. *Rhodochrosite*, on a pendant or in donut form, nourishes the heart. *Morganite* reduces the impact of trauma and *Citrine* restores joy, while *Black Tourmaline* will help her to forget the experience. These crystals can be used by day and also by night, tucked under her pillow.

Bed-wetting
Urinating while asleep

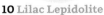

10 Lilac Lepidolite

15 Rose Quartz

26 Red Jasper

If your little girl wets the bed but not seriously enough to require medical intervention, put a piece of *Lilac Lepidolite* under her pillow to calm her nervous system. Add *Rose Quartz*, on a necklace, bracelet or in donut form, to improve the quality of her sleep. Psychologists say that bed-wetting is caused by anxiety or some transient fear. It is best to discuss it with your little girl, to reassure her and to restore her confidence by giving her a *Red Jasper* crystal that she can wear during the day, perhaps on a pendant if she so wishes.

Shyness
Helping her break out of her shell

3 Blue Chalcedony

30 Turquoise

9 Lapis Lazuli

Children are quite often shy. A mother may also have suffered shyness in the past. If that is true of you, talking about it with your little girl can reassure her. Explaining your own past or present difficulties will strengthen the mother–daughter bond. What sorts of things prompt her shyness? Try to find out from her how she feels. Does it happen in front of certain people? Or in specific situations, possibly recurring ones? Knowing the answers will help you choose the crystal best suited to her. *Turquoise* on a pendant or necklace (worn next to the throat) will allow her to speak up, using the right words to assert herself. *Blue Chalcedony* is more suitable if the little girl is naturally reserved or inhibited, because this crystal will relax any tightness she feels in her throat and encourage her to speak freely. *Lapis Lazuli*, worn on a pendant, in donut form, on a necklace or bracelet, also makes it easier to communicate.

Sense of loss
When she feels abandoned

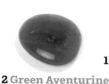

2 Green Aventurine

15 Rose Quartz

5 Chrysoprase

30 Turquoise

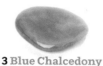

3 Blue Chalcedony

As a little girl grows up she finds herself facing different types of separation, such as leaving school friends or a teacher she particular likes or, within the family, the loss of a grandparent or a pet. She may experience it as abandonment and suffer grief. Whether worn on a necklace or pendant, *Green Aventurine*, which comforts grief, and *Rose Quartz*, which calms, will both bring great relief. *Chrysoprase* will help her to accept change and should be placed in her pillowcase or worn on a pendant. These three crystals will restore the emotional security she may have lost. It is important for the child to talk about her feelings. *Turquoise*, on a pendant, and *Blue Chalcedony* will help her express her sorrow. Depending on her age, Turquoise encourages expression through drawings, colour and mime, while Blue Chalcedony will help her to talk about matters close to her heart.

Fatigue
How to restore a child's vitality

21 Amber

22 Copper

17 Ruby

7 Red Garnet

In towns and cities, as well as our own homes, we're subjected to many types of pollution. It is well known that lack of sunshine, sea air or fresh air can weaken children. To strengthen a child's natural defences, choose *Amber* on a necklace or in donut form, or *Copper*. Unlike Amber, Copper should only be used occasionally.

Ruby boosts and restores energy, but should be removed as soon the tiredness has gone away, especially if a child is naturally fiery. Lastly, *Red Garnet* has an energizing effect and can be worn on a pendant, in donut form, on a necklace or a bracelet.

Colds
Get out the handkerchiefs!

11 Malachite

23 Emerald

1 Amethyst

5 Chrysoprase

9 Lapis Lazuli

For mothers, winter, with its continuous trail of colds and associated symptoms, from runny noses and painful ear infections to sore throats, can seem never ending. *Malachite*, on a pendant, necklace or in donut form, has a beneficial effect on the nose, throat and ears. Its beauty will enchant a child who loves the colour green. It also treats sore eyes, as does *Emerald*, which should be worn on a pendant. For headaches, use *Amethyst*, but for sinus pain *Chrysoprase* (on a pendant) is preferable, especially if the child has weak lungs. *Lapis Lazuli* clears congested respiratory tracts.

Falls
Knocks, bruises and bumps

22 Copper

25 Hematite

11 Malachite

24 Fluorite

4 Orange Calcite

A child is naturally active: she runs, she rides a bike, and falls and sprains are inevitable. These can be soothed with *Copper*, which is effective for treating sprains or pain. Attach a piece to the painful area. *Hematite* reduces bruising and can be worn on an anklet, around the wrist, on a pendant or kept in a pocket. *Malachite* has similar properties. The little girl should decide for herself which stone she prefers. When treating sprains, *Fluorite* strengthens cartilage. *Orange Calcite* encourages the absorption of calcium to strengthen bones after a fracture.

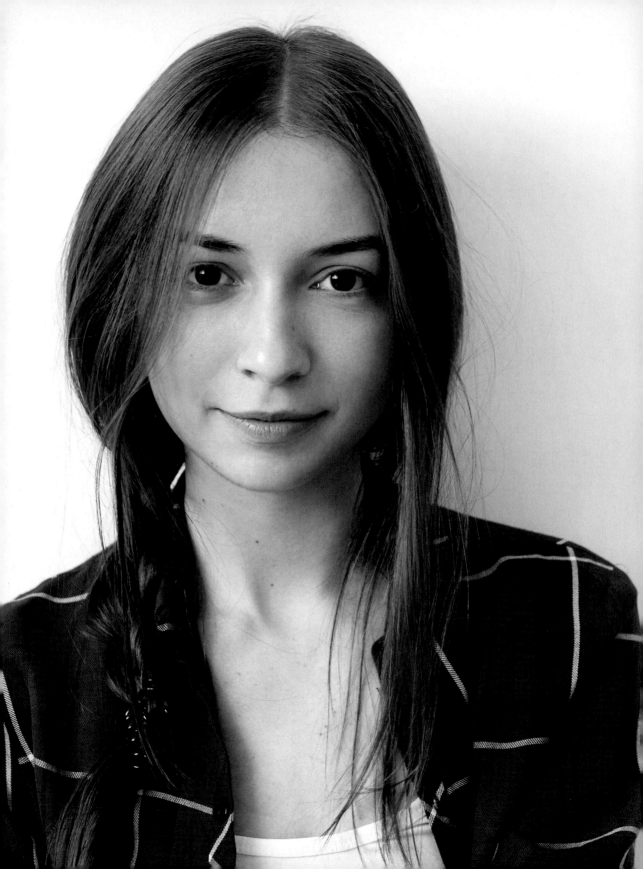

Healing crystals
for teenage girls

Childhood ends … and that period called adolescence begins. It starts at around 13 years at the onset of menstruation and ends around the age of 18. The disruptive hormonal and physical changes occurring at this time both contribute to a personality change. The teenager learns to assert herself and live with oestrogen and progesterone, the new hormones circulating in her system, which will soon make her an independent woman.

Let's take a look at the crystals that can help to navigate through all of this!

Puberty

The hormone surges that define the menstrual cycle are often painful and destabilizing - physically, psychologically and emotionally. Adolescence can be a tricky time for mothers who are often fearful - with or without cause - but it can also enhance a mother-daughter relationship if both continue to trust and talk openly to each other. Periods start and will continue until your daughter reaches the menopause. Her body will change. Her breasts will fill out. Body hair may be a problem. Skin gets greasy and spotty and hair will be lank as a result of overproduction of sebum. Yet, it is now that she is gradually transformed day by day from ugly duckling to the magnificent swan she will be as an adult woman.

Mood swings
Leave me alone!

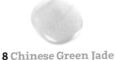

8 Chinese Green Jade

4 Orange Calcite

6 Citrine

19 Imperial Topaz

Orange Calcite helps a teenager overcome her sad moods. It encourages her to stop complaining and keep smiling. It gives her self-confidence and helps her to put things into perspective. This crystal can be kept in a pocket, or worn on a pendant, a necklace or bracelet. It can also be slipped under her pillow at night. *Citrine*, too, will put a smile on her face. This crystal transforms a bad mood into a happy one and can be used in the same way as Orange Calcite. *Imperial Topaz* encourages awareness. Life is so much simpler when you stop wearing a sad face. There are daily tasks to be done and being in a bad mood is not going to change that. A teenager can wear this crystal on a pendant or necklace. She can also use a mixture of these crystals together, choosing the ones that appeal to her at a particular time.

Or perhaps she would rather stay moody? It's up to her to decide. Most importantly, let her choose and test the crystals that attract her. For the sake of her mother and the entire household, she should just experiment and stay positive. *Chinese Green Jade* will help her to find the right balance. It encourages healthy introspection so that she can better understand herself. It will develop her judgement and enable her to maintain solid moral principles to get through life's stormier times. It is a crystal of honesty and wisdom that will help her to speak out justly and truthfully. It conveys its quality of loyalty to whoever wears or carries it. It is also said to attract good fortune and is believed to be a potent symbol of luck. It can be used in donut, pendant, earring or bracelet form.

Teenage tantrums
When tempers flare

11 Malachite

1 Amethyst

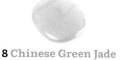

8 Chinese Green Jade

15 Rose Quartz

18 Sapphire

A piece of *Malachite* can calm the sometimes inexplicable outbursts that occur at this time. It helps a teenager to keep her self-control. She can place it in her pillowcase at night or, if she prefers, she can wear the crystal around her neck on a necklace, pendant or in donut form. Malachite will encourage her to open her heart and will help her think carefully about what she says to those around her. Conversations can and must be calm, rather than heated exchanges where either she or other people get angry.

Malachite also encourages good judgement. *Amethyst* will help her to control her temper. It can be worn on a necklace, earrings, bracelet or pendant. If some of her reactions seem surprisingly extreme, *Chinese Green Jade* and/or *Rose Quartz* can be used together with Amethyst. *Sapphire* will reassure anxious teenage girls who seek to dominate by screaming or shouting. It can be worn on a necklace, a pendant or a bracelet, or put under her pillow or carried in a jeans pocket or in her bra.

Sleep
Getting a good night's rest

Lapis Lazuli encourages sleep. Each night, your teenager can place this crystal on her forehead and let herself be soothed by soft, calm music. When she gets drowsy, she can slip the stone under her pillow. *Amethyst* banishes sleepless nights. It is best for her to wear a necklace made up of both stones at night or to put them under her pillow.

9 Lapis Lazuli

1 Amethyst

Headaches & the teenage mind

Ease the pressure

9 Lapis Lazuli

10 Lilac Lepidolite

1 Amethyst

11 Malachite

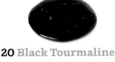

20 Black Tourmaline

Getting wound up about a problem can often trigger headaches. *Lapis Lazuli* will help a teenager pinpoint the causes of her concerns. It will enable her to look at the reality of a situation coolly and dispassionately. She should place it on her forehead to stem the flood of worrying thoughts. It will calm her mind and she will become more objective and positive. Alternatively, she can place it on the nape of the neck or under her pillow. *Lilac Lepidolite* is also calming and brings serenity. To enjoy that essential peace of mind, this crystal, too, should be placed on the forehead. Consider *Amethyst* as well; it banishes sad thoughts and sows the seeds of positivity. It controls over-emotional feelings and hypersensitivity caused by

fluctuating hormones. For this, it can be worn on a necklace, in donut form or placed under her pillow. *Malachite* relieves headaches caused by hormone surges or by an excessive intake of fatty or sugary foods. It has a regulating and calming effect on the liver and gall bladder. It can be worn on a necklace, pendant or slipped under her pillow. Finally, *Black Tourmaline* neutralizes the harmful electromagnetic waves emitted, for example, by computers, televisions and mobile phones, which can cause headaches. A beautiful large Black Tourmaline crystal must be placed in a room where electronic machines are used. It is also worth remembering that electronic screens in a bedroom will make it harder to fall asleep.

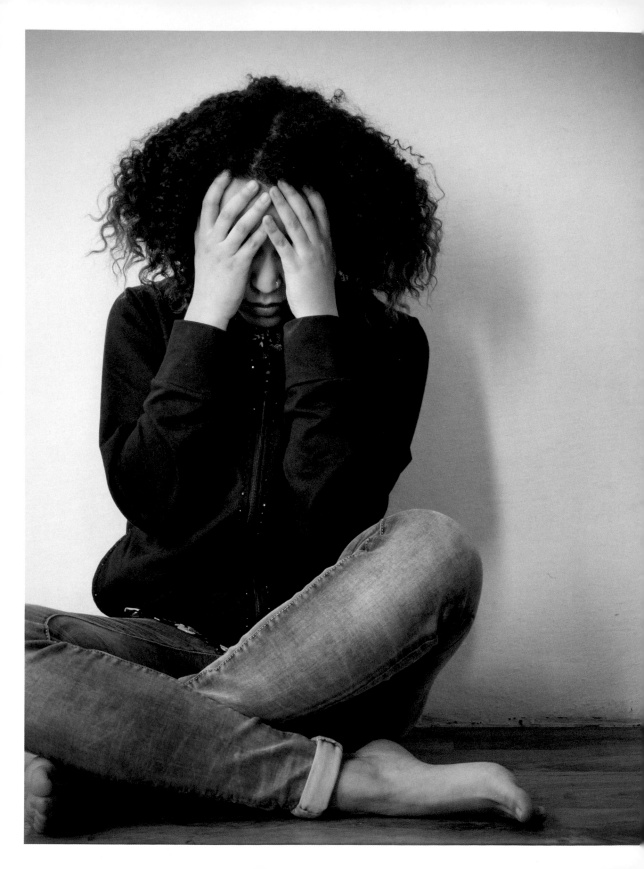

Sadness
A flood of emotions

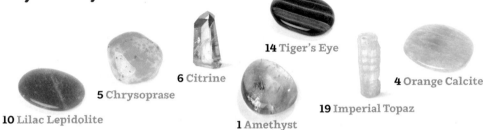

14 Tiger's Eye

6 Citrine

5 Chrysoprase

10 Lilac Lepidolite

4 Orange Calcite

19 Imperial Topaz

1 Amethyst

Lilac Lepidolite relieves sadness, encouraging serenity and peace. It balances fragile emotions. The teenager should keep it under her pillow at night and wear it on a pendant or necklace during the day. Together with *Chrysoprase*, it will give her the desire to move forward. With further reinforcement from *Citrine*, she will rediscover the joy that lies dormant within her. This stone will bring her a ray of sunshine. It will awaken laughter and light-heartedness, and can be worn in donut form, on a necklace, as earrings or a bracelet. *Tiger's Eye* rebalances oversensitive emotions, especially if she feels excessive empathy. During the menstrual cycle, when her emotions are high, she may absorb everyone else's sadness. This crystal should be worn in donut form over her heart. *Amethyst* encourages positive thinking. It relieves conscious and underlying sadness. *Orange Calcite* offers that hopeful ray of light that helps everything to work out well. It supports serenity, encouraging us to spread its calm among all those around us. It can be worn on a necklace, as a ring, bracelet or earrings. Lastly, *Imperial Topaz*, worn on a necklace or pendant, brings joy, enabling her to live in harmony.

By getting in touch with her reactions and feelings, she will be able to experience the sense of achievement which the world of healing crystals puts within her reach. Adopting a positive attitude and maintaining it will be important throughout her entire life.

Isolation
Feeling alone in the world

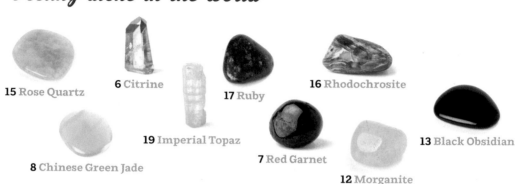

15 Rose Quartz   **6** Citrine   **17** Ruby   **16** Rhodochrosite

19 Imperial Topaz   **13** Black Obsidian

8 Chinese Green Jade   **7** Red Garnet   **12** Morganite

As a first step, the teenager should wear a flat donut of *Rose Quartz* close to her heart or in her bra. It will convey its power to comfort. She will be able to communicate with the crystal and thank it for being there. *Chinese Green Jade* will help her accept the situation and set her thinking, 'Why am I alone? Do I want to meet people?' And, if the answer is yes, 'What will new relationships mean for me?' *Imperial Topaz* supports and consoles someone who feels abandoned. It shows her the positive side of her situation by reassuring her that it is only temporary. There will be plenty of new encounters! Meeting others is a way of finding yourself. Next, the teenager could record her introspective feelings in a notebook. She should also talk to her school or college nurse or to one of her teachers or to her family doctor. Human beings aren't made to live alone. *Citrine* will help her to develop the confidence she lacks. Together with *Black Obsidian*, it will encourage her to recognize underlying fears and will give her the power to overcome them. *Red Garnet* will fill her with courage. *Ruby* can also help by encouraging strength and perseverance. *Morganite* can relieve that vague sense of unease that makes her feel sad. *Rhodochrosite* will comfort her and support her when she is disappointed in love.

Sensitivity
How to stop getting upset about nothing

14 Tiger's Eye

26 Red Jasper

3 Blue Chalcedony

30 Turquoise

Tiger's Eye makes a teenager more forgiving when she faces criticism or malicious gossip. This crystal will teach her how to look beyond negative comments and see the situation from a different, more positive viewpoint. It can be worn in donut form, on a necklace, earrings or bracelet. *Red Jasper* moderates emotionally charged words. It will make her quick-witted enough to put things into perspective. *Blue Chalcedony* will show her how to respond. *Turquoise* will make her more thick-skinned and able to ignore wounding criticism. These stones can be worn on a necklace, pendant, in donut form, tucked into a bra or on a bracelet. To banish bitterness and oversensitivity, there's nothing better than experiencing positive emotions such as gratitude, laughter and joy. The teenager can implement this positive psychology by writing down the positive responses she experiences with the crystals in her special notebook. This may take a few minutes but will bring clear benefits.

Addiction
When teenagers become 'hooked'

1 Amethyst

9 Lapis Lazuli

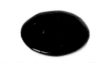

20 Black Tourmaline

Some young girls – those who are emotionally fragile or unsure of themselves – may have a tendency to copy other people. They follow the crowd or, to try and look more grown-up, may drink alcohol or smoke, or may compensate by overeating. Others escape reality by shutting themselves off in the virtual world of video games, where they can lead their lives at one remove from reality. In such cases, *Amethyst* can help the withdrawal process and *Lapis Lazuli* will calm extreme urges. *Black Tourmaline* further protects against electromagnetic radiation, provided it is regularly cleaned and recharged.

A desire for freedom
Dear Parents, I'm off!

9 Lapis Lazuli

7 Red Garnet

17 Ruby

20 Black Tourmaline

27 Magnetite

Teenagers feel an intense need to break out of the framework of everyday life and to taste freedom. Seeking out thrills and extreme excitement in all sorts of forms is one of the urges experienced at this age. *Lapis Lazuli* can instil clear thinking and help a teenage girl face up to reality. It can be worn around the neck, in donut form, on a pendant or a necklace. *Red Garnet* will help her keep her feet on the ground. It will help her make sensible choices when she is tempted to be over-impulsive. It can be worn on an anklet or kept in her pocket. *Ruby* can help a teenager build and maintain her vitality. It will influence her judgement and allow her to channel excessive energy appropriately. This crystal will help her see how to make good decisions that guide her in life.

It will encourage her to behave respectfully. Ruby can be used in the same way as Red Garnet. *Black Tourmaline* helps to anchor her in everyday life. It can be invaluable for certain types of addiction, such as social media or online video games. It enables a teenager to distance herself from an addiction and become aware of reality. It can be worn on a necklace, in donut form, on a pendant or bracelet, or it can be kept in a pocket. *Magnetite* encourages realignment. It indicates the path forward to well-being. It will help a teenager meet the right people at the right time. If it is supported by positive thoughts, it will attract positivity. It can be worn on the ankle, on the wrist or around the neck.

Intuition
Encouraging perceptiveness and creativity

9 Lapis Lazuli

26 Red Jasper

27 Magnetite

20 Black Tourmaline

1 Amethyst

Many young girls are not aware that they are potentially more intuitive and creative during their menstrual cycle. *Lapis Lazuli* helps a teenager to benefit from this throughout the day and night. She can put it under her pillow or wear it on a necklace, pendant or earrings. It will bring inspiring dreams and creative ideas. By day it can be used together with *Red Jasper* for keeping ideas grounded in reality and finding a way of acting on them. Putting plans into action will enable her to discover a sense of achievement. Red Jasper can be worn on a necklace, pendant or in donut form. *Magnetite* attracts creative ideas and lifts the potential barriers that might hold her back, such as self-doubting questions, like 'Why am I failing?' or 'How am I going to manage?' *Black Tourmaline* helps projects to take root and brings them to fruition. It can be worn as a pendant or in donut form between the neck and the heart area. *Amethyst* will help her to discover her own spirituality.

Call to action
Making dreams come true

27 Magnetite

20 Black Tourmaline

17 Ruby

7 Red Garnet

When *Magnetite* is worn on a pendant, dreams are acted on and then achieved. It is very useful to write down plans and projects in a notebook and re-read them on a regular basis. Little by little, the teenage girl will see that everything around her is taking shape in the most natural way, as Magnetite attracts positive situations. *Black Tourmaline* encourages awareness. It helps her to determine what sort of life she wants to lead as an adult. What profession will she choose, for example? *Ruby* gives projects momentum even when they're long-term plans. It imparts a life force and an unwavering will. *Red Garnet* inspires action. It makes us live life rather than dreaming.

Acne & greasy hair
Reducing sebum production

23 Emerald

22 Copper

21 Amber

29 Orange Moonstone

During adolescence, the sebaceous glands produce too much sebum; skin become spotty and hair becomes greasy at its roots. The hormonal cycle is usually the cause (with a significant peak before a period); overly fatty or rich food may also be to blame. *Emerald* helps to dry up and heal spots. To use it for this purpose, she should simply place one or more clean crystals in the jar of face cream or cleansing lotion that she uses. If Emerald is also worn on a necklace, pendant or earrings, this will strengthen its effect. *Copper* has the

same properties, so can be used similarly. *Amber* relieves inflamed skin and helps to regulate sebum secretion. *Orange Moonstone*, in an orange to greyish shade, will balance fluctuating levels of oestrogen and progesterone. A reduction in oestrogen production is what triggers a period, while the secretion of progesterone activates ovulation and, during adolescence, is also responsible for producing acne. Orange Moonstone can be worn on a necklace, pendant or earrings, or placed under a pillow.

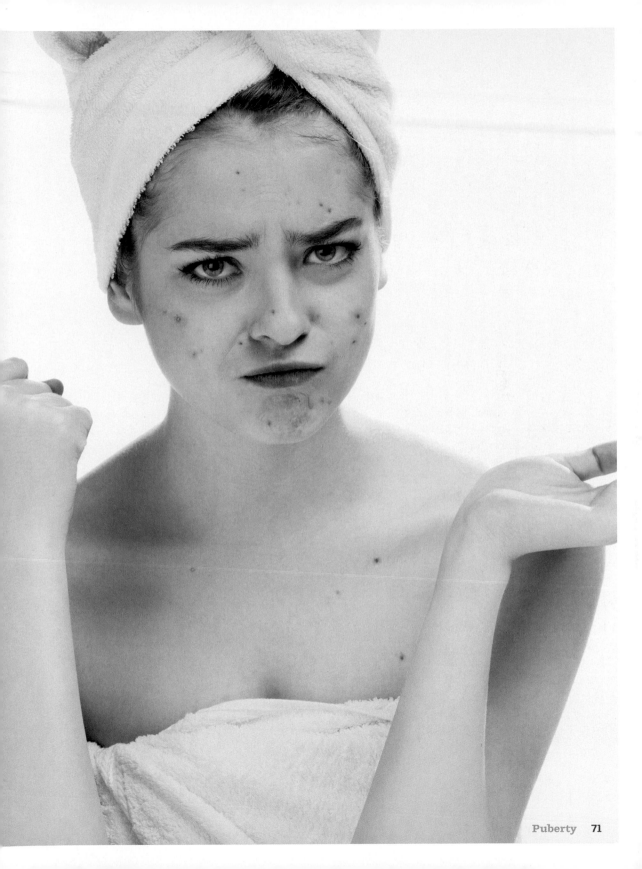

Femininity
Developing her charm and charisma

28 Freshwater Pearl

5 Chrysoprase

6 Citrine

A girl must realize that she has her whole life ahead of her for romantic relationships. Many boys prefer girls to look natural. Make-up should show her at her best but not transform her into a sophisticated adult. To enhance her attractiveness, *Freshwater Pearls* can guide her intuitively towards more feminine clothes. They will inspire her to show off her hair in a flattering style or help her highlight some other stunning feature. They should be worn on a pendant or choker. *Chrysoprase* will let her dare to assert her femininity. It will make her want to pamper and take care of herself. Forget leggings and shapeless T-shirts! This crystal will be useful for girls who want to accept and acknowledge a slim waist and a developing chest. It will encourage her to wear a skirt, a dress or very 'girly' printed T-shirts. And it can be worn in a very feminine way on a necklace, pendant or earrings. If a teenage girl is in need of self-confidence, *Citrine* is worth considering. It helps an adolescent take her place and be respected within her peer group. The crystal will make her joyful and positive. On a necklace or pendant, it has a flattering effect. It can also be worn in the form of a bracelet or earrings.

Vitality
Getting in shape

27 Magnetite

5 Chrysoprase

14 Tiger's Eye

24 Fluorite

7 Red Garnet

Doing some kind of sport is essential for physical, emotional and mental well-being. Because of their fluctuating moods, teenage girls tend to try one sport after another: 'I'd like to try that …'/'I don't want to go any more …'. OK, girls, but now is the time to get moving! A teenager should choose a sport she likes and stick with it. *Red Garnet* encourages enthusiasm and competitiveness. It can be worn in donut form or on a pendant placed over the solar plexus, together with *Magnetite*, which will help her do well while avoiding muscular cramps. *Chrysoprase* will enable her to achieve a specific objective; she can put a flat stone in her pocket or slip it into her bra. Girls who are less physically strong should carry a *Tiger's Eye* crystal in each hand while running, to help develop their muscles (and this stone also prevents stitch). For other sports it can be worn on an anklet. So, off to the playing field and no more excuses! And that includes growing pains, which are no reason to avoid exercise. And if ever she suffers a sprain, *Fluorite* can be attached or placed over the injured area.

Cellulite
Fluid-retention problems

Because of its draining effect, *Freshwater Pearl* helps to prevent weight gain. It is during adolescence that the body takes on the shape of the future woman. Cellulite begins to form during puberty. Freshwater Pearl prevents cellulite caused by water retention from appearing on the tops of the thighs, on the buttocks or around the abdomen. (See also Vitality: Getting in shape, above.)

28 Freshwater Pearl

Self-confidence
Building self-esteem

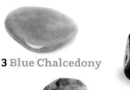

3 Blue Chalcedony

27 Magnetite

30 Turquoise

24 Fluorite

7 Red Garnet

19 Imperial Topaz

6 Citrine

4 Orange Calcite

An adolescent girl may sometimes need to feel supported and encouraged. *Blue Chalcedony* will give her grace of movement that will make her appear more feminine. When she wears the crystal on a pendant, her gestures will be more confident. With the help of *Turquoise*, she will be able to express herself in a gentle way. This crystal can be worn in donut form, on a necklace or as earrings. *Magnetite* will strengthen her confidence and concentration and will help her shine. Carrying this crystal in her pocket, or wearing it in donut form on a pendant, will work wonders. The stones can also be used at night, tucked under her pillow. If the teenage girl feels the need to belong to a group, she should perhaps consider *Red Garnet*.

It will help her listen to others and find her place within the group. It also aids concentration. A Red Garnet necklace is an impressive piece; keeping the stone is her pocket is more discreet. *Fluorite* is an excellent companion during revision or exam time, as it encourages reflection. There is a wide choice of colours as the crystal may be green, blue or purple, or also multicoloured or veined. Fluorite jewellery comes in the form of necklaces, pendants, bracelets or earrings. *Orange Calcite* builds self-confidence little by little. *Citrine* brings joy and the desire to take up challenges. *Imperial Topaz* will free her from malicious gossip and give her the courage to begin again.

Making an anklet

Materials
The crystals can be bought in a specialist outlet, at mineral fairs or online (see page 27); the other materials can be found in a handicraft shop.

• Nylon thread, fishing twine or elastic thread
• Flat pliers
• Pair of scissors
• Fastener
• Crimp beads (also called 'squeeze beads')
• Beads of your choice (here Amber is shown)

1 Take the thread and pass it through the small Amber stones.

2 Finish it with a crimp bead or tie a knot. Make a bracelet large enough to slip on to your ankle without breaking the thread.

Alternative method: make an anklet with a fastener and have a few fine beads hanging from it so it doesn't feel uncomfortable with socks.

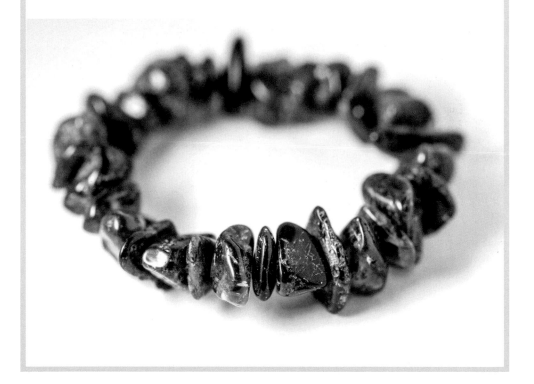

Menstruation

Periods are perfectly natural. Every
28 days or so, they remind a female that
she has the ability and the opportunity
to create new life if she decides to do so.
Emotional sensitivity or extreme events
can sometimes upset the cycle or cause
irregularities. The duration of periods
can also vary, as every woman is different.

Stomach pain
Painful periods

21 Amber

5 Chrysoprase

14 Tiger's Eye

22 Copper

Menstruation can be physically and mentally disruptive, especially for teenagers whose cycle is not yet regular. If periods are painful, it is a good idea to lay two flat pieces of *Amber* on the lower stomach and hold them in place with a plaster. *Chrysoprase* relieves any pains around the genital area; a crystal in donut form can be worn there during the night. *Tiger's Eye* can be used in the same way to relieve pelvic congestion – pain from dilated veins, often around the ovaries. Two round, ball-shaped pieces of *Copper* can also be used to relax the ovaries in mid-ovulation. Using small circular movements, roll both pieces together over the area to relieve the pain. It works!

Tiredness
Feeling worn out

25 Hematite

7 Red Garnet

17 Ruby

Hematite treats that extreme tiredness that a female may feel during her period. Menstruation involves the loss of varying amounts of blood and this crystal, because of its significant iron content, has a regenerating effect on haemoglobin, the protein molecule in red blood cells. The crystal can be put in a jeans pocket or worn on a pendant or an anklet (see page 75).

Red Garnet stimulates blood circulation. Its action relieves the pain, heaviness and sometimes swelling in the lower limbs that may occur during periods. Teenage girls who feel creative could make themselves two anklets with these crystals. *Ruby* boosts blood circulation and restores vitality. It can be worn on the ankle, around the wrist or around the neck.

Nervousness
Boosting blood circulation

22 Copper

7 Red Garnet

17 Ruby

25 Hematite

Many teenage girls and women become a little nervous and fearful during their menstrual cycle because of the blood lost, which the body has to replenish. *Copper* regulates body heat. It creates a sense of warmth and has a revitalizing and regenerating effect on blood, preventing anaemia. It also stimulates the liver, ensuring that iron is properly absorbed. When necessary, holding a piece of Copper in each hand can be helpful. It can also be kept in a pocket or handbag so that it's always within reach. *Red Garnet* also warms the body by stimulating blood circulation and can be used in the same way as Copper. *Ruby*, too, has a warming effect if a crystal is slipped into each pocket. *Hematite* will likewise restore body heat.

Painful breasts
Easing swelling and tenderness

Amber reduces the swelling that causes breasts to be tender during periods. Wear it on a necklace or put a piece of Amber in each bra cup. *Tiger's Eye* relieves the pain and can be used in the same way. *Copper* will reduce any kind of stabbing pain. It is best to choose a flat piece of Copper for this. However, a round ball-shaped piece of Copper can be doubly effective when applied with a circular movement: roll it around the breasts in the shape of a figure of eight.

21 Amber

22 Copper

14 Tiger's Eye

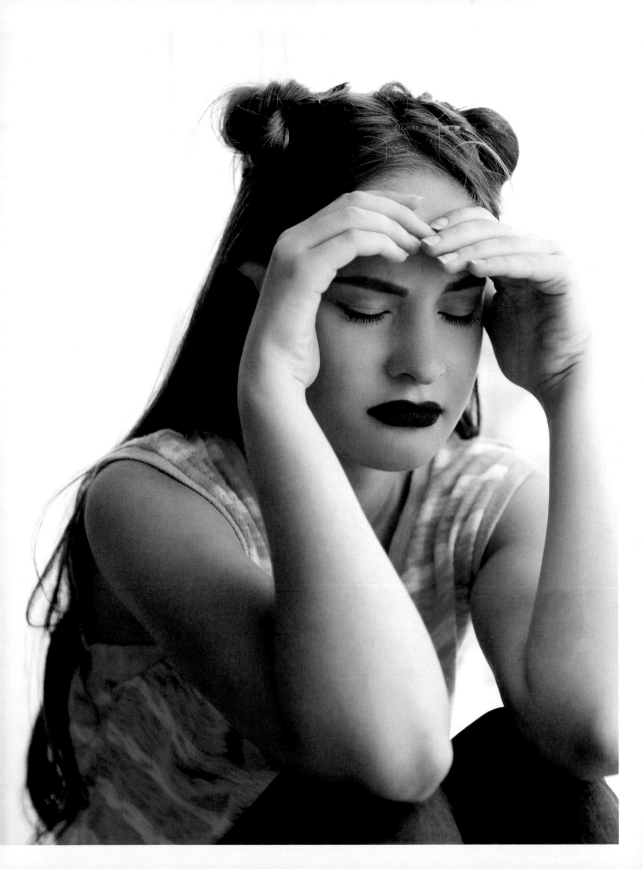

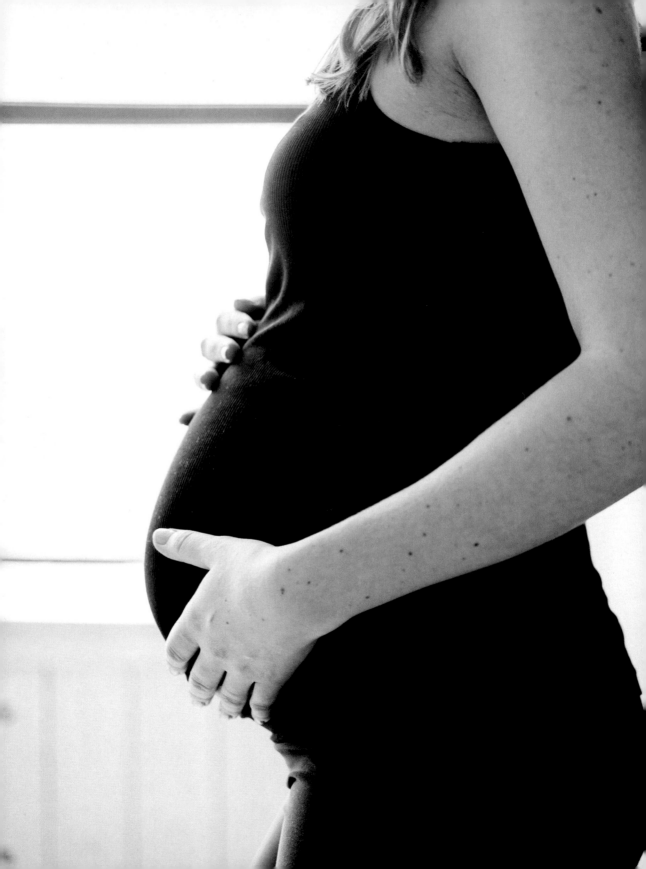

Healing crystals
for women and mothers-to-be

When a girl's teenage years end, her endocrine system – the glands that secrete hormones into her circulatory system – will be well established. As a woman she will live with a regular hormonal cycle for the next 30 or so years. The chaotic world of work will confront her with all sorts of changes to which she will have to adapt. Her heart will beat to the rhythm of love. Her children will raise her adrenaline levels, surprising her with the unexpected and sometimes with their absence.

Let's take a look at the crystals that can help to navigate through all of this!

At work

Working life can give a woman important financial independence. The world of work also offers the chance to learn about all sorts of issues that - like certain people - can sometimes be quite surprising. But work and health are inextricably linked. Between the drudgery of a job that feels like forced labour and one that inspires our passion lies a whole spectrum of possibilities. Let's look at the best ways of living through this important time and finding personal fulfilment.

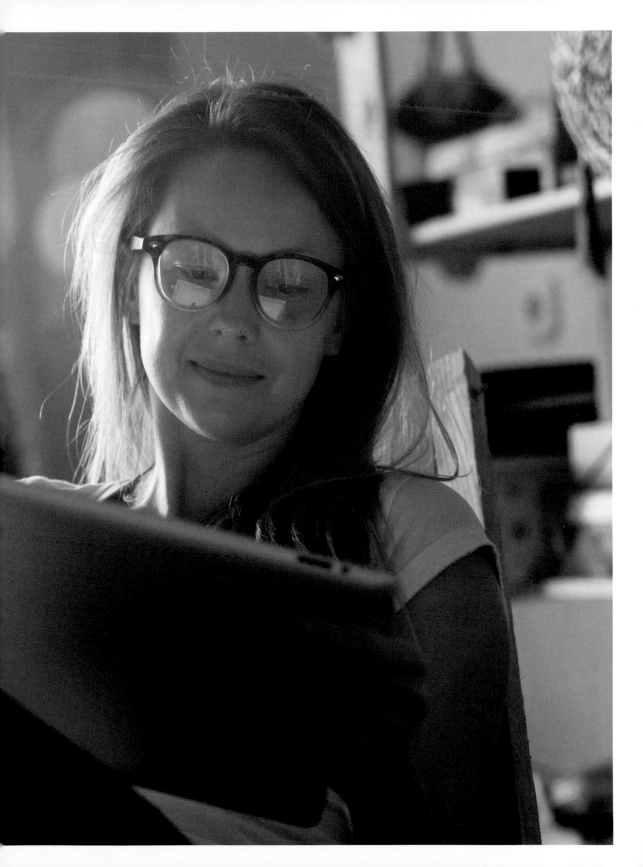

Motivation
A great job!

14 Tiger's Eye

4 Orange Calcite

17 Ruby

7 Red Garnet

18 Sapphire

Tiger's Eye helps you to maintain and achieve the goals you set yourself. It can be worn on a necklace, in donut form, on a pendant or a bracelet. *Orange Calcite*, used in the same way, helps you feel confident and capable of carrying out the different tasks required. *Ruby* is supportive when the hierarchy at work creates a volatile environment. Wear it dangling gracefully from your neck or around your wrist. *Red Garnet* encourages you to take back control of your working life. It can be worn as an attractive choker or bracelet. A working woman should also consider *Sapphire*, which offers stability. This, too, can be worn on a necklace or bracelet.

Guilt
Accepting that you're not perfect

8 Chinese Green Jade

7 Red Garnet

9 Lapis Lazuli

Days are only 24 hours long. Which of us hasn't wished they could be longer to enable us to complete a busy schedule? Women – often unconsciously – feel guilty for not being able to do all the work they want to do or ought to do in a day. Wearing *Chinese Green Jade* on a bracelet or necklace will be a help and support. It will encourage you to be fair to yourself, to know your limits and to accept them. *Red Garnet* is energizing. Together with *Lapis Lazuli*, it provides insight. This crystal will let you analyse the causes of these feelings of guilt and trace them back to their roots, sometimes in the distant past. Does this guilt come from your mother's or father's side? Or from siblings, your partner or 'false' friends?

Jealousy
When emotions at work are running high

14 Tiger's Eye

13 Black Obsidian

18 Sapphire

30 Turquoise

1 Amethyst

8 Chinese Green Jade

Tiger's Eye drives away malicious gossip in the workplace. It can be worn on a necklace, in donut form, on a pendant or bracelet. *Black Obsidian* helps you to realize that wounds must be healed to enable you to develop and flourish. It is best worn close to the heart or on the neck, or slipped into a pocket or under your pillow. *Sapphire* clears emotional blocks and calms frayed nerves.

It should be worn preferably on the neck, or else around the wrist. *Turquoise* will guide you towards good communication and truth. It can be used in many ways – worn on a necklace, in donut form or on a bracelet, or placed under your pillow. *Amethyst* calms excessive, out-of-control emotions, while *Chinese Green Jade* tempers envy.

Author's note

Catherine I have given a number of workshops where the theme was guilt. (These were my Irisame workshops, where photographs are used to evoke emotions.) The participants often complained of localized pain around the shoulders or lungs. Sadness and anger were among the emotions mentioned. I could tell that the burden of guilt was a weight on their shoulders and that it brought a sadness that was felt around the lung area (just as outlined in traditional Chinese medicine).

Exercise Find a place where you can be alone and remain still and calm for about 30 minutes with a Lapis Lazuli necklace or crystal in your hand. Think of nothing and open your mind to insights. You can also sleep while holding the necklace or placing the crystal under your pillow. Ask your inner self what might be the cause of your sense of guilt. Repeat the exercise each evening until you get a response. When you are silent or resting at night, dreams and insights will come to you. It is useful to make notes and to re-read them, as it sometimes takes time to understand messages from our unconscious.

During the exercise, painful sensations may be felt in parts of the body, such as the throat, the back or the stomach. It is interesting and useful to link the emotion experienced to where it is felt. This area will be different for different people.

At the end of the exercise, you should write down in a notebook what you experience in terms of increased energy, well-being and lightness. These are the best indication that the exercise has been a success!

Communication
Promoting teamwork

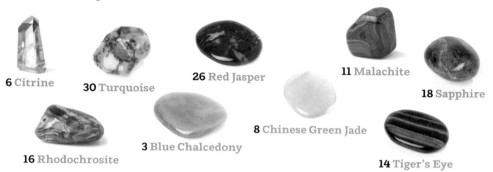

6 Citrine
30 Turquoise
26 Red Jasper
11 Malachite
18 Sapphire
8 Chinese Green Jade
16 Rhodochrosite
3 Blue Chalcedony
14 Tiger's Eye

In an office, communication can be cold and impersonal, and exchanges bitter and dehumanizing. *Rhodochrosite* improves teamwork and maintains good relationships within the group. Decisions will be just, considered and flexible. In discussions, *Turquoise* improves understanding and boosts mental skills. This crystal, which favours balance, helps keep words gentle and considerate when it is difficult to be conciliatory. In this way, it forges links in a group that shares the same objectives. *Citrine* helps everyone to find their place and pull together. *Red Jasper* builds team spirit. Each of these crystals can be worn on a pendant, in donut form, on a necklace or bracelet.

If the atmosphere becomes difficult and oppressive, *Blue Chalcedony* will bring calm and reflective thinking. It allows you to take a stand and to consolidate your position in a gentle way; wear it on a necklace, bracelet or pendant. *Chinese Green Jade* lets you avoid stormy outbursts. It could be useful to add other crystals. If the outburst has occurred, it is advisable to wear a calming *Malachite* necklace to help you to reconnect with yourself. Lastly, to help you get your ideas together and react appropriately, focus on *Tiger's Eye*, which gives you courage and a powerful but not excessively loud voice. No longer will you be swayed by others! You can put an end to those dirty tricks which insidiously upset the balance and hurt people. Lastly, *Sapphire* worn on a necklace or a pendant will help you to focus on your goals and reconnect with yourself.

Anger
When tempers explode

11 Malachite

1 Amethyst

2 Green Aventurine

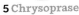

5 Chrysoprase

14 Tiger's Eye

What can you do when emotional tension rises to a dangerous level? How can you calm seething anger? How do you control it? Keep a piece of *Malachite* with you in a pocket of your handbag and hold it when an over-emotional outburst could hurt others – and above all yourself. Getting angry too often is harmful to health! *Amethyst* calms a negative, aggressive mood. *Green Aventurine*, worn close to the heart, encourages you to make the fairest decisions in a difficult situation. *Chrysoprase* helps you to find an effective fallback position; anger is pointless if the other party enjoys provoking you. Some women are naturally too passive! They should focus on *Tiger's Eye*, which offers courage and helps you to make your voice heard without raising it excessively. This tiger is ideal for timid women who are downtrodden at work.

Frustration
Annoyances and disappointments

9 Lapis Lazuli

15 Rose Quartz

6 Citrine

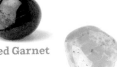

7 Red Garnet

14 Tiger's Eye

5 Chrysoprase

30 Turquoise

Whatever the cause of the disappointment, *Lapis Lazuli* will stem the flood of negative thoughts that can submerge you. You should simply place the crystal on your forehead and leave it there for as long as necessary. *Rose Quartz* will relieve frustration if you wear it close to your heart; it can be easily hidden in a bra. *Citrine* helps you to look forward with confidence. It can be kept in a pocket or worn on a pendant, in donut form or on a bracelet.

Red Garnet gives you the ability to recover and bounce back, and can be used in the same way as Citrine. To help you move on, consider *Chrysoprase*, which allows you to accept the situation and put it to rest. It, too, should be worn close to your heart. *Tiger's Eye* will let you forge ahead and enlarge your circle of professional contacts. *Turquoise* should be used with it. The two stones can be worn together on an anklet or a bracelet.

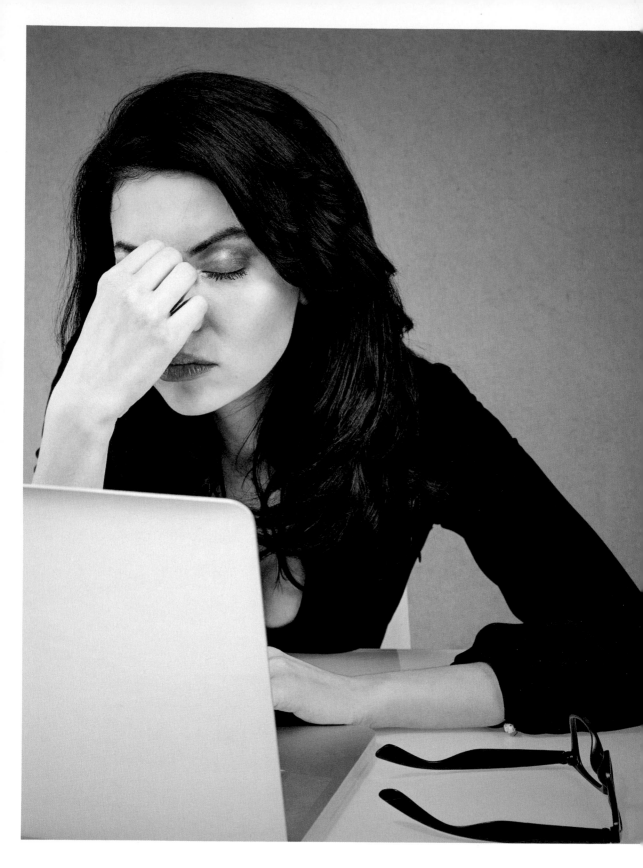

Organization & burnout
Stop feeling overloaded

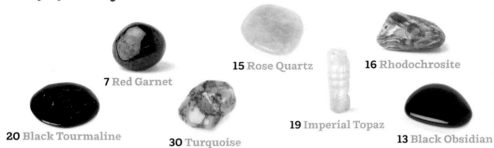

7 Red Garnet

15 Rose Quartz

16 Rhodochrosite

20 Black Tourmaline

30 Turquoise

19 Imperial Topaz

13 Black Obsidian

Black Tourmaline could successfully organize the work of a government minister – and even prioritize the tasks! Don't forget it. This crystal is ideal for rediscovering your sensitivity and responsiveness, as it balances the dark 'yin' principle. It can be slipped into a pocket, worn close to the heart or put under a pillow. *Red Garnet* energizes and maximizes the little strength remaining at the end of marathon days. It can be used in the same way as Black Tourmaline. *Turquoise* develops the organizing abilities that every woman has. Keep it with you day and night in any form you like. Invigorating *Imperial Topaz* will help you to confront everyday stress; it is best worn on a bracelet. In our daily routine, the unexpected can seem like a wild beast that has to be tamed. When faced with unforeseeable events and the emotional tension they bring, consider *Rose Quartz*, which will help you keep an open heart and mind. It will stop you from sinking into bitterness or anger. *Rhodochrosite* has much the same effect. It will give you an energy boost if you are tired. These crystals should preferably be worn next to the skin on a necklace, pendant or in donut form.

Black Obsidian brings a sense of where the happy medium lies. This idea draws on the notion of yin and yang, which corresponds with the duality of everything: for instance, the white and the black, and yang activity and ying repose. The two sides are constantly changing. The priority is to avoid excess and maintain balance. Black Obsidian reorients us. Beware of burnout – literally burning up energy until it is exhausted. It is essential to be able to draw a line, even though it is true that life sometimes overloads us with responsibilities that have to be taken on whatever the cost.

Dismissal

Keeping active and bouncing back

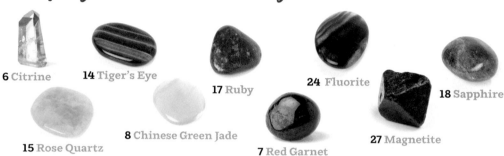

6 Citrine

14 Tiger's Eye

17 Ruby

24 Fluorite

18 Sapphire

15 Rose Quartz

8 Chinese Green Jade

7 Red Garnet

27 Magnetite

Rose Quartz and *Chinese Green Jade* will help you to accept the situation. The first crystal will do this by opening up your mind to other future possibilities; the second, by giving you the wisdom to come to terms with your current state. Both crystals can be slipped into a pocket or worn around the neck. In this situation, *Citrine* helps you maintain your moral values. A flat stone can be placed in a bra or on the stomach.

Tiger's Eye will help you to get back on track and take up further studies or a training course. Keep it in your pocket. What job would you really like to do? *Red Garnet* encourages you to achieve things you have so far failed to do. *Fluorite* aids concentration when worn close to the throat. *Magnetite* attracts work that will meet your criteria and match your individual abilities. It can be kept in a pocket, worn next to the heart or placed under your pillow. It takes courage to find a new job, and *Ruby*, when kept deep in your pocket, will make you brave. When we need advice or a decision, aren't we often told to 'sleep on it'? When placed under your pillow, *Sapphire* will encourage reflection and be a guardian angel.

Resignation
A conscious choice

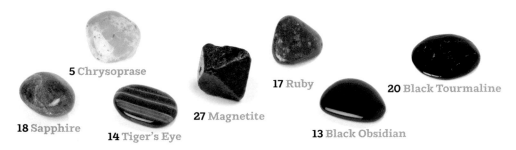

5 Chrysoprase

18 Sapphire

14 Tiger's Eye

27 Magnetite

17 Ruby

13 Black Obsidian

20 Black Tourmaline

Because of something that has happened, you've decided to resign. How nice it would be if you'd done so because you wanted to get involved in charitable work or join some aid organization. Sadly, people often resign because they've had enough, following a series of difficult incidents. Before leaving, *Sapphire* will encourage you to jot down a list of the jobs you would like to do. That will enable you to bounce back and apply for jobs you haven't tried before. The crystal should be slipped under a pillow at night, as ideas and inspiration often come at this time. You must remain hopeful and *Chrysoprase* is good for indicating the path to new beginnings. It is best worn on a pendant, in donut form, on a necklace or bracelet. *Tiger's Eye* encourages you to roll up your sleeves and move forward.

It can be kept in a pocket or worn around the neck. Consider *Magnetite*, as it could attract the job that perfectly matches your individual skills. Wear it close to your heart or tucked into a pocket. *Ruby* supports decision-making and supplies the courage required to quit a current job and find a new one. It can be worn on a necklace, pendant or bracelet. However, it is not advisable to wear it at night, as its effect can impair sleep. *Black Obsidian* brings a clear awareness of the situation experienced. *Black Tourmaline* encourages calmness before making decisions. These crystals can be worn on a necklace, in donut form, on a pendant, or bracelet, and can also be kept close by you at night. Do not forget to chart your progress in your notebook.

Falling in love

That first encounter is magical: you're in love and your view of the world changes. You're full of joy, confidence and hope. Your heart is flooded with light and ready to explode. Reason seems to vanish for a while; you're on cloud nine and it feels so good. Make the most of it, as reality will return soon enough. Those initial whirlwind feelings can sometimes change, bringing disappointment. No matter; it is essential to love, as all incurable romantics would agree.

Meeting
When Prince Charming comes calling ...

27 Magnetite

28 Freshwater Pearl

19 Imperial Topaz

7 Red Garnet

18 Sapphire

30 Turquoise

The ideal man can be anywhere; each woman has her own individual selection criteria, based on both physical features and character traits. Some may dream of finding a cordon bleu chef or a DIY expert with exceptional skills; others will prefer relaxed couch potatoes or tough sports types.

In fairy tales the prince sweeps up the beautiful maiden and carries her away on his charger. Today, that prince could well be the postman, someone who delivers your pizza or groceries, a neighbour or perhaps the person you have met via the screen of your mobile or laptop. These days a loving partner may come from anywhere. The best advice is to make a list of your main interests, whether cooking, sport, reading, films, dance, walking or something else, and then the type of life partner who might be compatible. This is a useful exercise. Sometimes it's preferable to socialize in places where people go specifically to meet each other and then just let it happen – while discreetly carrying *Magnetite* in your pocket to attract any susceptible hearts that are out there. *Freshwater Pearl* will help you to find your perfect match. They say you catch more flies with honey than vinegar, so try *Imperial Topaz*; masculine energy will succumb to its charms, especially if it is worn around a pretty neck. *Red Garnet* kept in a pocket is more likely to attract female energy. *Sapphire* will help launch a good relationship and both partners should wear it on a pendant or necklace. *Turquoise* encourages you to explore the emotional intelligence of your other half. Wear it in the same way as Sapphire.

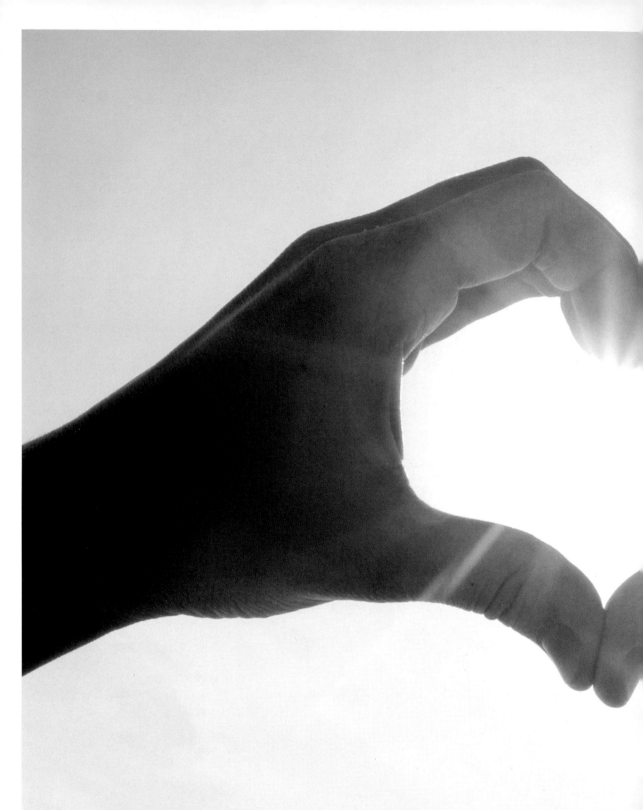

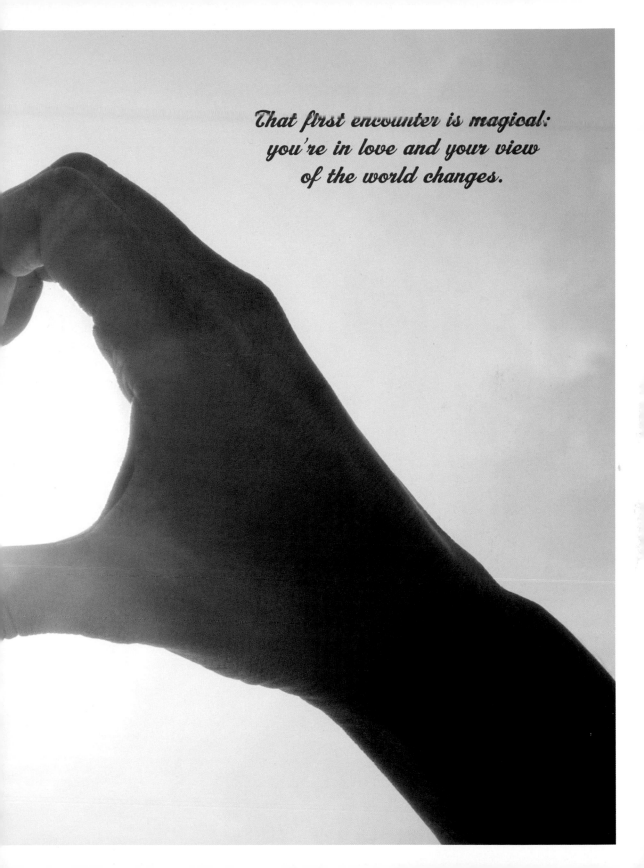

*That first encounter is magical:
you're in love and your view
of the world changes.*

Betrayal
When love strays

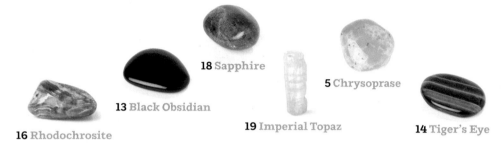

18 Sapphire

13 Black Obsidian

5 Chrysoprase

16 Rhodochrosite

19 Imperial Topaz

14 Tiger's Eye

To start with you could try *Rhodochrosite* to relieve the heartache of betrayal and to help put things into perspective. This crystal also arouses sensuality, which lies dormant within everyone. You could slip *Black Obsidian* into your pocket or under your pillow to understand what attracted you to a womanizer. Sometimes we have these seemingly incomprehensible emotional blockages deep within our hearts, which compel us to accept the unacceptable. In such cases, *Sapphire* can whisper a solution. It works well when placed under your pillow. *Imperial Topaz* conveys wisdom and brings gentleness and patience into a couple's private life. It should be worn against the throat and close to the navel. *Chrysoprase* lets you move forward bit by bit towards a decision that will give you – or restore – a sense of well-being. *Tiger's Eye* offers the necessary push to make you take the plunge. Happiness is within the grasp of everyone. This crystal will give you the courage to make decisions in these circumstances. It can be worn simultaneously on a necklace, in donut form and on a bracelet, or it can be placed under your pillow.

Break-up (not your choice)
Mourning your love

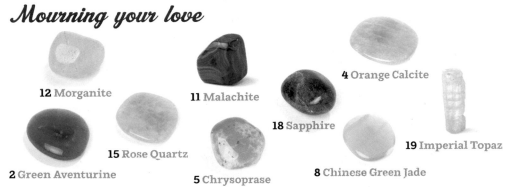

12 Morganite

11 Malachite

4 Orange Calcite

18 Sapphire

19 Imperial Topaz

15 Rose Quartz

2 Green Aventurine

5 Chrysoprase

8 Chinese Green Jade

Green Aventurine helps you accept the break-up of a relationship and lay it to rest. *Rose Quartz* will support you through this emotional turmoil. If these stormy times have shaken you up, *Morganite* will comfort you and also let you forgive yourself. It calms hearts that are devastated by remorse and sadness and sets them on the path to recovery. These crystals can either be worn together or separately on a necklace, in donut form, on a pendant or bracelet, or tucked into a bra or under a pillow. *Chrysoprase* allows you to calmly go forward alone. *Orange Calcite* gently but surely restores self-confidence. It can be used together with the four previous crystals. *Sapphire* will encourage you to be kind to yourself. It makes it easier to take a close look

at yourself, which is essential for understanding why certain similar situations may occur again and again. *Chinese Green Jade* encourages you to be true to yourself without getting lost in a labyrinth of emotions. It is highly effective when worn in donut form against the heart, but can just as easily be used in other ways. *Imperial Topaz* tends a wounded heart by opening your mind to wisdom and optimism. It is best worn close to the chest or on the stomach, or slipped under your pillow. When grieving, we may be tempted to indulge in our worst friends – chocolate, butter and cream. If, as a result, you suffer gall-bladder pain, use *Malachite* and attach it to the painful area; the length of time required will depend on how much you've consumed and on your age.

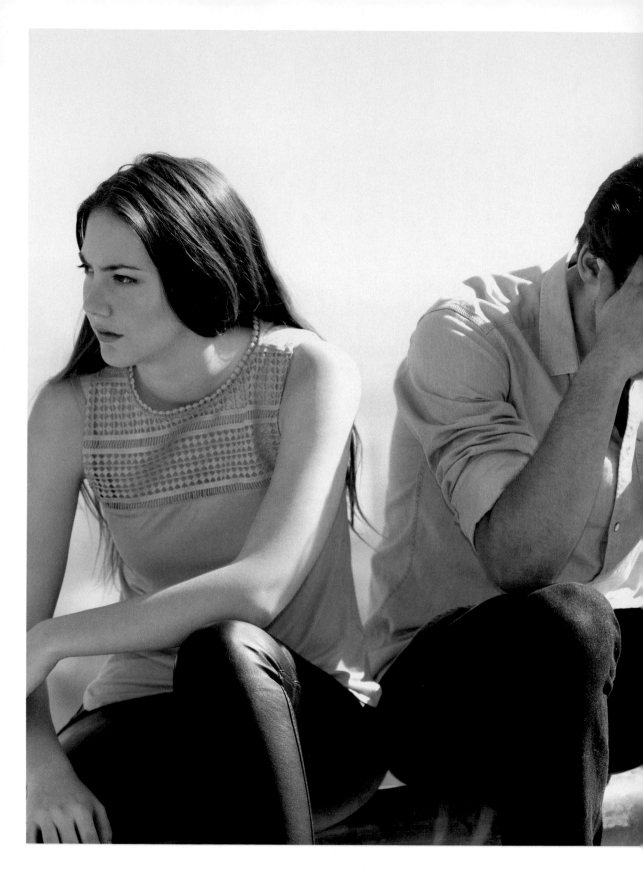

Break-up (your choice)
A time for self-reflection

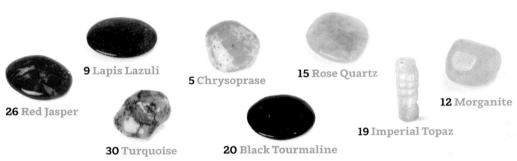

26 Red Jasper

9 Lapis Lazuli

5 Chrysoprase

15 Rose Quartz

30 Turquoise

20 Black Tourmaline

19 Imperial Topaz

12 Morganite

You have to take your courage in both hands to make the break. But then a new companion – guilt – appears! Making a fresh start is never easy. *Red Jasper* will help you to remain objective about the decision you have taken. If the situation has reached this point, it is because the relationship was no longer working. *Lapis Lazuli* helps you breathe when you're overcome by the spiral of events. *Chrysoprase* allows you to keep your objectives in mind so you can move on without looking back. *Black Tourmaline* relieves any guilt by lifting your mood. *Rose Quartz* calms the emotional stress caused by a stream of memories. *Morganite* brings peace of mind when break-ups mark the end of a difficult relationship. *Turquoise* will guide you on a new path and can renew anyone's optimism. Lastly, *Imperial Topaz* will shed light on what the future without your partner looks like.

Fertility & infertility

Being fertile begins with a healthy lifestyle and regular check-ups with your gynaecologist. If your doctor considers your reproductive system to be in good working order and you are well balanced mentally and emotionally, fertility should come quite naturally.

Sexuality

Discover or relearn the Kama Sutra to break up your routine!

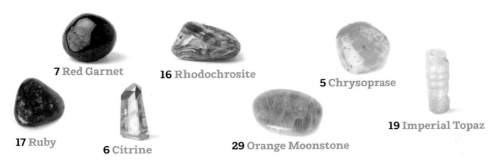

7 Red Garnet   **16** Rhodochrosite   **5** Chrysoprase

17 Ruby   **6** Citrine   **29** Orange Moonstone   **19** Imperial Topaz

Meeting someone reliable and stable may take time. Over the years, sexual desire can sometimes become a vague memory. Now is the time to rekindle it! A *Ruby* awakens both partners to sensual caresses. Wear this stone on a necklace, a pendant or an ankle chain. *Red Garnet* encourages a woman to develop her sensuality. When worn on the waist, neck and wrists, it stimulates sexuality. *Rhodochrosite* also encourages sensuality, but with a touch of naughtiness to spice up your love life. *Citrine* encourages playfulness, especially if placed on the navel. It could also be worn as a necklace, in donut form, on a pendant, a bracelet, or just slipped into a pocket. *Chrysoprase* will revitalize your ovaries, encouraging them to produce healthy eggs. This crystal brings a breath of fresh air, a feeling of renewal and change. It stimulates vitality. In the evenings, before going to bed, starting from the first day of your period, place one stone on each ovary. This crystal will also help you to release and dissolve feelings of guilt or shame … as long as your current partner is patient. *Orange Moonstone* rebalances the menstrual cycle and encourages fertility. Place it on the ovaries at night whenever you feel the need. *Imperial Topaz* encourages partners to be tender and more caring outside their intimate sexual relationship – perhaps by presenting an unexpected rose, a surprise breakfast, or placing a love note on a pillow or on the car windscreen. In this way, the crystal nurtures desire. It should be worn close to the heart.

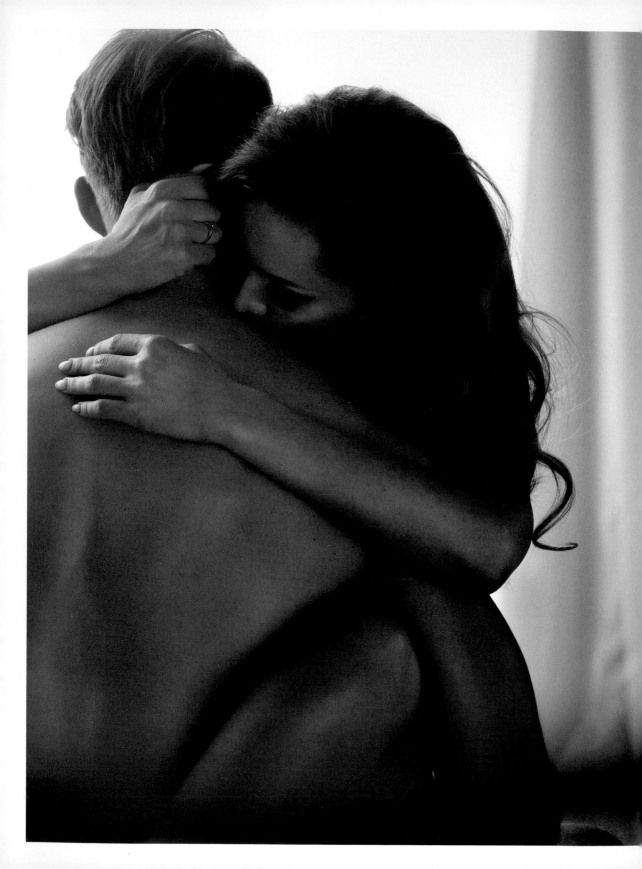

Infertility & fertility treatment
Loving care and perseverance

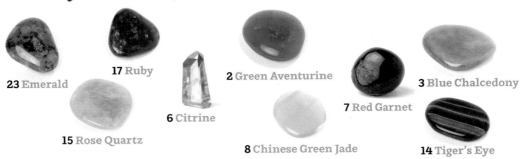

23 Emerald

17 Ruby

6 Citrine

15 Rose Quartz

2 Green Aventurine

8 Chinese Green Jade

7 Red Garnet

3 Blue Chalcedony

14 Tiger's Eye

When infertility becomes apparent, and medical intervention is required, the following selection of crystals can very helpful.

The list of obstacles that must be overcome when undergoing fertility treatment is a long one: keeping your confidence and patience intact, overcoming distressing examinations and ensuing disappointments, following instructions to the letter, putting up with the side effects of hormonal treatments, supporting a partner who's feeling the strain … However, it's not all negative; even if this period is intense and filled with a roller coaster of emotions and difficulties, at the end of the road there is happiness and the joy of giving life. To remain patient and hopeful, keep a *Rose Quartz* crystal with you (for calmness) or wear *Chinese Green Jade* (for patience) as a necklace, a pendant or in donut form. To combat fatigue, you can also wear this crystal on a bracelet during the day, or else place a *Ruby* on the kidney area to boost energy levels. A necklace of *Red Garnet* should be worn all the time, to maintain energy, vitality and strength.

The route to conception via fertility treatment can really shake up a couple's relationship to the point where they may for a while get tired of each other. Red Garnet can restore harmony, by awakening sexual desire and encouraging more frequent and fulfilling sex. Combine it with love-strengthening *Green Aventurine*. Add *Citrine*, too, which brings joy. These crystals can be worn on a necklace, pendant or in donut form. We suggest keeping them in the bedroom, either under the sheet or your pillow.

At different times, and for hormonal or many other reasons (for example, while you're undergoing the many necessary examinations), you may feel angry inside. Chinese Green Jade softens this sense of bitterness. *Emerald* reinforces the desire to create a family, while *Tiger's Eye* revives the determination to succeed in your stated objective. If it's just a simple passing irritation, wearing *Blue Chalcedony* should be enough. Its gentleness will calm and comfort you. These minerals should be worn on a necklace, in donut form or on a bracelet.

Pregnancy

Pregnancy is a miraculous process – the development and birth of a child in nine months. Some women may suffer various physical and emotional problems as a result of hormonal changes. The following pages explain which crystals a mother-to-be should keep with her at this time.

Author's note

Nathaëlh When I was pregnant, I practised 'haptonomy' (a holistic bonding therapy) without knowing it. From the first trimester of my pregnancy, I would press my hand against my lower abdomen and move it around very gently. In the second trimester, I felt something pressing from the other side. I don't have words to describe the emotion I felt at that instant. The baby's father and grandmother joined in. Separately or together, we put our hands on my abdomen and my unborn baby recognized our touch. I would say to him: 'Hello little one, are you sleeping?' Very often, he would seem to be rubbing against my hand. After six and a half months, he seemed to recognize voices. One after the other, we would say, 'Where is Grandma?' And he would move and snuggle under my mother's hand. Close to the delivery date, he would push more forcefully against my hand. After the birth, during Shantala sessions (Indian massage for babies), my baby blew bubbles and gurgled with happiness much earlier than other babies. From early infancy, my son gained an emotional maturity, which made him more independent, for instance, when we left him with a childminder or when he went to nursery. It is a magical experience and I would recommend it to anyone.

Morning sickness
Feeling nauseous

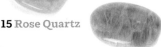

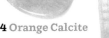

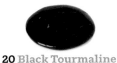

15 Rose Quartz

4 Orange Calcite

20 Black Tourmaline

6 Citrine

29 Orange Moonstone

19 Imperial Topaz

Vomiting is the result of hormonal changes and usually starts in the morning. So it is a good idea to link up with *Citrine* early on. This Quartz mineral will bring relief and make you feel more comfortable. It works best when the stone, in donut form or tumbled, is placed on the stomach when you go to bed and during the day. If the sickness is caused by emotional problems, we suggest wearing either a *Rose Quartz* bracelet or necklace, whichever is most suitable, for at least three nights, combined with a small *Orange Moonstone* placed under the pillow, or worn on a necklace, pendant or bracelet, or in donut form or tumbled. *Orange Calcite* combats nausea, while *Imperial Topaz* relieves gastric acidity. It is worth noting that, at the very early implantation stage, *Black Tourmaline* placed just below the navel helps the embryo adhere to the wall of the uterus.

Backache
Ease the strain

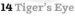

22 Copper

16 Rhodochrosite

11 Malachite

18 Sapphire

14 Tiger's Eye

If you're suffering from lower back pain, place a donut-shaped piece of *Tiger's Eye* on the area to relieve the tension. You can, if wished, combine it with *Rhodochrosite* if the pain is caused by emotional stress. *Copper*, *Sapphire* or *Malachite* can also ease the pain as a result of their copper content.

State of mind
Overcoming doubts and uncertainties

9 Lapis Lazuli

17 Ruby

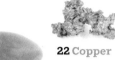

3 Blue Chalcedony

22 Copper

18 Sapphire

27 Magnetite

Your brain is in turmoil, full of doubts and questions. Nervous exhaustion sets in. *Lapis Lazuli* will calm your thoughts and stop them spiralling; wear it on a necklace. *Ruby* restores mental balance and may be more suitable, depending on your emotional state. *Blue Chalcedony* worn on a necklace or in donut form will help you to express all the thoughts and fears that come into your mind. It will also sweep away sad and negative ideas and change the way you think. When you get worked up, a small piece of *Copper* will calm your nerves. Hold it in your hand or wear it on a bracelet. *Sapphire* and *Magnetite* work together. It is a good idea to note down the differences you experience with them.

Sleep
Enjoying peaceful nights before the baby arrives

17 Ruby

6 Citrine

26 Red Jasper

22 Copper

1 Amethyst

Sometimes, as soon as you wake up, you feel tired and as if you haven't slept at all during the night. Depending on your emotional state at the time, choose between the following five crystals. *Ruby*, on a pendant, boosts energy levels. It gives you the desire and the strength to tackle things despite your tiredness. A necklace of *Citrine* will put you in an excellent mood. *Red Jasper* on a bracelet or in donut form will tone your muscles and improve circulation. *Copper* will eliminate toxins, provided you drink enough liquids; it can be worn on a bracelet, necklace or in donut form. And *Amethyst* is always the uncontested queen of calm nights when worn on a necklace, in donut form, or placed under a pillow.

Compulsory bed rest
When you must ease off

25 Hematite

1 Amethyst

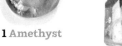

6 Citrine

4 Orange Calcite

19 Imperial Topaz

There are times when you will get impatient, especially if the doctor orders bed rest. You may have to lie down for several days or several months, in which case choose *Hematite* to avoid problems associated with prolonged inactivity. This time can be an excellent opportunity to get in touch with your unborn baby, the ideal moment to practise what is known as 'haptonomy' (see page 104). Via the power of touch on her abdomen, the mother-to-be (and her partner) will be able to contact and stimulate the baby during its time in the womb, producing reactions that help to build a loving relationship. For this, *Amethyst* is

the crystal of choice, as it will help you to bond more strongly with your baby. It brings wisdom and balance and is spiritually uplifting. If time passes slowly and your confidence flags while you're lying there immobile, *Citrine* will reassure you with the certain knowledge that the baby will arrive. This crystal will lighten your mood and raise your confidence levels. *Orange Calcite* similarly keeps you hopeful. This crystal is gentler and less stimulating than Citrine. Use *Imperial Topaz* when you feel tired and gloomy. These crystals can be worn as you wish on a necklace, in donut form or on a pendant.

Appetite
Too big or too little?

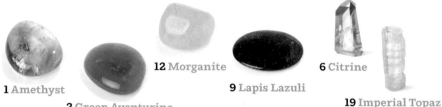

1 Amethyst

2 Green Aventurine

12 Morganite

9 Lapis Lazuli

6 Citrine

19 Imperial Topaz

Grandmothers often maintain that during pregnancy you should eat for two! Of course, they are thinking of a double portion of fresh vegetables or fruit. Nowadays, however, it's often sugary treats – sweets, cakes or chocolate – or salty ones, such as crisps and savoury snacks, that tempt the appetite. One typical craving is for strawberries with lots of sugar. But if either the mother or the baby put on too much weight, the birth can be difficult. *Amethyst* can effectively control pregnancy cravings. It can be worn on a bracelet, necklace, in donut form or carried in a pocket. *Green Aventurine* steers your food choices towards natural produce. *Morganite* will free you from guilt, while *Lapis Lazuli* can rein in an excessive appetite.

Some women don't eat enough because they fear they will retain all the weight gained during pregnancy. That is wrong thinking. With a balanced diet, then breastfeeding, getting back to an active life and a little sport, everything will return to normal. *Citrine* will stimulate the appetite. *Imperial Topaz* offers the wisdom to understand that the food consumed by a mother-to-be contributes to the well-being of her foetus. These crystals can be worn or carried in any form as desired.

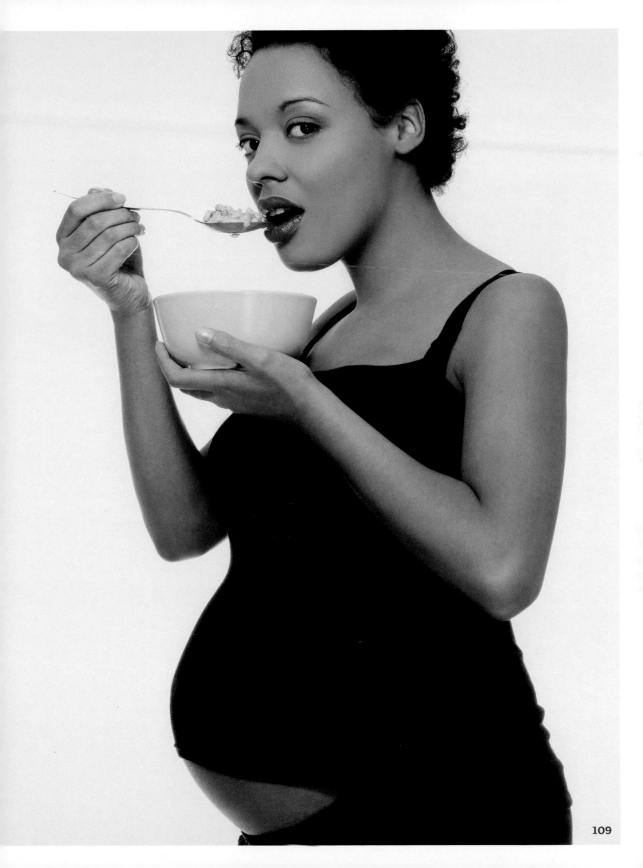

Aching legs & cramp
Relaxing the body

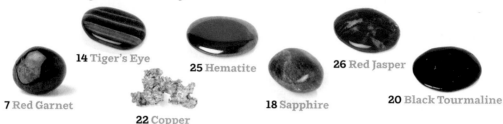

14 Tiger's Eye

25 Hematite

26 Red Jasper

7 Red Garnet

22 Copper

18 Sapphire

20 Black Tourmaline

Wearing anklets of *Red Garnet*, which stimulates blood circulation, will relieve painful legs. Slipped into your pocket, *Tiger's Eye* soothes the sciatic nerve and eases muscle cramps. Placing *Copper* on the skin or in a pocket also reduces the pain. With its vigorous warming effect on blood circulation, *Hematite* combats night cramps. *Sapphire* offers support in the tense time before the birth, which can seem interminable. It can be worn or used in whichever form you prefer. A piece of *Red Jasper* under the bed covers will get rid of muscle cramps. This crystal also stimulates blood circulation. *Black Tourmaline* can be used in the same way as Red Jasper. It has a significant magnesium content which helps to relax muscles.

Gestational diabetes
An unwelcome guest

6 Citrine

11 Malachite

22 Copper

Diabetes often develops at the end of pregnancy. The pancreas is effectively having to secrete twice as much insulin as normal – for mother and baby. If your diet is healthy, the stimulating effect of *Citrine* can regulate your blood sugar levels. Because of its copper content, *Malachite* and, of course, *Copper* itself will help to detoxify the body. In addition, remember to drink frequently to eliminate any excess sugar.

Anaemia
Depleted red blood cells

Even if the anaemia is mild, the suggested crystals are no replacement for medical treatment, of course. They will simply improve your sense of well-being. Wear *Hematite* on a pendant, in donut form or on a necklace. *Ruby* on a pendant does its bit by stimulating blood circulation. *Red Garnet* acts in the same way and is best worn on the ankle or wrist.

25 Hematite

7 Red Garnet

17 Ruby

Acne
Going back to adolescence

2 Green Aventurine

23 Emerald

12 Morganite

22 Copper

It's tedious for a mother-to-be to face a problem she first overcame in teenage years. For this problem, we suggest you look back at the relevant section (see page 70) and consider these four crystals: *Green Aventurine* infused in water can be used to dab on the spots, as can *Emerald*. Orangey pink *Morganite* relieves acne problems and *Copper* is also effective.

Constipation & haemorrhoids
Moving food gently through the system

Even with a balanced diet including plenty of vegetables and fibre, constipation can still occur. At night, wear *Red Jasper* in donut form or place the crystal on the painful intestinal area. If haemorrhoids develop, find a small piece of tumbled *Sapphire* and put it close to where you feel the pain.

26 Red Jasper

18 Sapphire

Cystitis
Infections to avoid

22 Copper

11 Malachite

28 Freshwater Pearl

An infection can always occur; take care, and, while waiting for a doctor's appointment, place *Copper* or *Malachite* in donut form on the bladder area. *Freshwater Pearl*, which has a draining effect, is recommended for urinary problems as long as you drink plenty of water. Place it at the bottom of the glass or bottle of water you are drinking from.

Headache
Controlling your hormones

First, you should turn to *Amethyst* for help. Choose a deep purple stone and wear it preferably on a necklace. Amethyst is recommended when headaches are due to stress or tiredness. *Orange Moonstone* will soothe headaches that are caused by hormonal changes.

1 Amethyst

29 Orange Moonstone

Blood pressure
A roller-coaster time

1 Amethyst

18 Sapphire

26 Red Jasper

17 Ruby

7 Red Garnet

16 Rhodochrosite

5 Chrysoprase

12 Morganite

4 Orange Calcite

Morganite is a suitable healing crystal when a shock, such as bad news, causes your blood pressure to rise. *Rhodochrosite* calms troubled emotions. Wear it on a necklace, a bracelet or in donut form. *Sapphire* on a pendant also calms stress. *Amethyst* helps to regulate blood pressure, as does *Orange Calcite*. *Red*

Jasper encourages a normal blood pressure level. These stones can be worn as you wish. *Chrysoprase* also helps – wear it on a necklace or in donut form, as desired, and let the crystals work for as long as necessary. If your blood pressure is too low, wear a *Ruby* on a pendant. *Red Garnet* also boosts low blood pressure.

Acid reflux
Nervous stomach

6 Citrine

28 Freshwater Pearl

To relieve acid reflux, a crystal should preferably be placed on or attached to the problem area, always next to the skin. Because of its yellow colour, *Citrine* is linked to the digestive zone. It can be used day or night in tumbled or donut form whenever the burning sensation occurs. *Freshwater Pearl*, which is basically made up of nacre (the iridescent substance that coats the

inside of the mollusc's shell), relieves the pain of a nervous stomach and helps you to become aware of repressed frustrations. During pregnancy, a normally quiet stomach can become very noisy. This crystal prevents those unpleasant sounds by relieving gastric acidity. When you get an attack, use it by day or at night infused in a bottle or glass of fresh water.

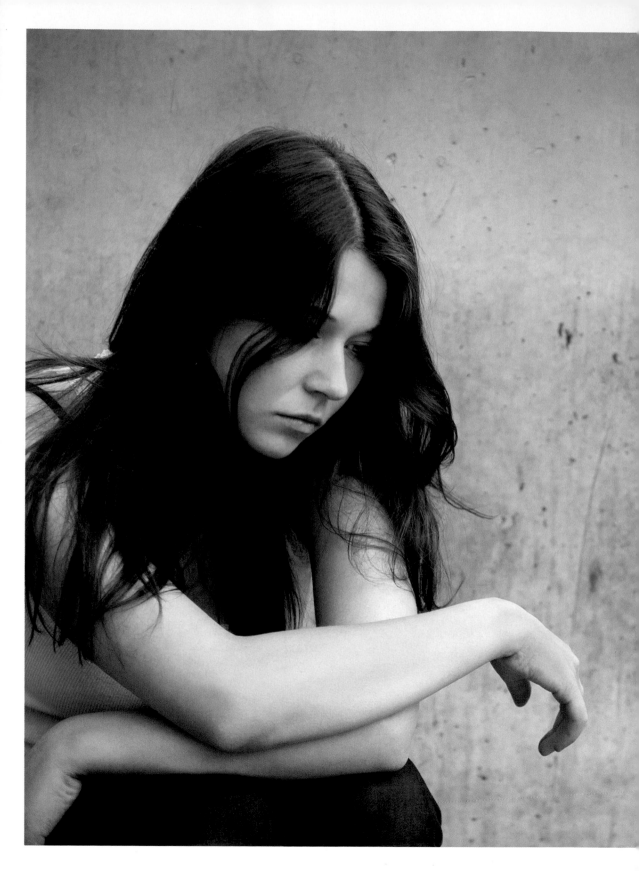

Facing pregnancy termination
Emotional issues

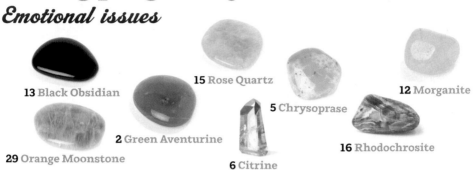

13 Black Obsidian

15 Rose Quartz

5 Chrysoprase

12 Morganite

29 Orange Moonstone

2 Green Aventurine

16 Rhodochrosite

6 Citrine

Abortion Whether it is your choice or necessary for medical reasons, an abortion will often trigger sadness, disappointment and feelings of guilt. Holding a piece of *Black Obsidian* in each hand reduces the cramping pains of such interventions. *Orange Moonstone* will also soothe pain following the abortion. Lay the crystal on the painful area or attach it. Wearing it day and night – on a necklace, pendant, bracelet or in donut form – will balance the hormonal system. Use it for as long as necessary, usually the two weeks following the abortion. *Green Aventurine* – also on a necklace, pendant, bracelet, in donut form, or under your pillow – provides support as you grieve, helping you to accept the situation. *Rose Quartz* comforts aching hearts and should be kept close to the heart on a pendant or tucked into a bra. Having it with you at night will bring calm. *Rhodochrosite* helps to release anguish. Place it on your chest. *Morganite* relieves deep emotional wounds. It brings forgiveness and understanding and is non-judgemental. Guilt goes away and compassion takes its place. It can be used or worn in the same way as the other crystals suggested here. *Citrine* brings joy and will shine when hung around your neck or on your wrist. *Chrysoprase* will give you the impetus to start over and also offers the hope of future success.

Rape Rape is a difficult experience to overcome – physically and psychologically – and it is advisable to consult a specialist. Quite wrongly, a victim may consciously or subconsciously feel guilty. *Green Aventurine* helps a victim come to terms with the past. By bringing insight into what has happened, *Morganite* relieves the trauma of the experience. Placed on the heart, it encourages compassion and boosts self-esteem. *Citrine* together with *Rhodochrosite* will bring light and chase the shadows away so that life can be lived calmly in the present. Both crystals can be worn together on a necklace or pendant.

Childbirth

The joy of being stuck on the couch, the delight of leaking urine when you carry something heavy or when you laugh, then kidney or pelvic pains ... These are sure signs that you will soon give birth. Many women believe that the experience of giving birth is the most beautiful and intense of their entire lives. While people talk about 'delivering' a baby, it's more a question of hard 'labour'. Happiness and pain come together. At the end there will be new life.

Backache
Relieving pelvic pain

18 Sapphire

22 Copper

14 Tiger's Eye

At last the baby's head is in position. *Sapphire* on a pendant will soothe the pelvic pains that occur several days before labour starts. *Copper* will relieve sciatica if that is still a problem. It also helps when contractions are felt around the kidneys and pain radiates into the lumbar area of the back. *Tiger's Eye* is also useful for combating backache.

Contractions
When labour begins

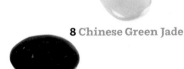

8 Chinese Green Jade

7 Red Garnet

17 Ruby

29 Orange Moonstone

20 Black Tourmaline

14 Tiger's Eye

Whether your waters have broken or not, contractions are starting. Holding pieces of tumbled *Black Tourmaline* in each hand will help you manage the pain of childbirth while you wait for an epidural. Similarly, *Chinese Green Jade* will give you the courage to bear the pain. If you feel cold between contractions, hold *Red Garnet*, which will help to warm you up. When it is a long labour, think of *Ruby*, to give you energy and make you feel less tired. To help you push, call on *Tiger's Eye*, which supplies the strength required as you imagine or visualize it. *Orange Moonstone* will help you to deliver your baby calmly.

Postpartum fatigue
Recovering your strength

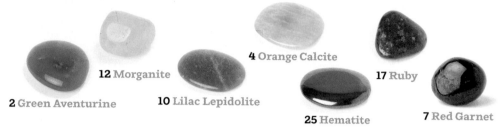

12 Morganite

4 Orange Calcite

17 Ruby

2 Green Aventurine

10 Lilac Lepidolite

25 Hematite

7 Red Garnet

Just after giving birth, some new mothers feel a profound sadness – akin to mourning the physical separation from the foetus and experienced almost like a bereavement. It is as if the symbiosis – their interdependency during pregnancy – continues in a purely emotional form. *Green Aventurine* helps to fill the void. *Morganite* relieves the tears shed in this loneliness. Little by little *Orange Calcite* fills the mother's heart with the sweetness and joy of the life she will share with her new baby. *Lilac Lepidolite* enables her to put things into perspective. *Hematite* is helpful when a new mother is convalescing after a postpartum haemorrhage. *Ruby* enables her to get back her strength if she feels exhausted. Finally, *Red Garnet* is useful for combating weariness and fatigue. These crystals can be worn on anklets or on the wrists, on a necklace, in donut form or on a pendant.

Breastfeeding
A very special closeness

15 Rose Quartz

1 Amethyst

18 Sapphire

21 Amber

5 Chrysoprase

9 Lapis Lazuli

When your breasts are one size larger, they can be painful: a piece of *Amber* in each bra cup brings real relief and also helps heal cracked skin. Once you start thinking about breastfeeding, a whitish *Rose Quartz* crystal will help the milk to come in. *Chrysoprase* provides support when the time comes for the baby to be weaned.

Amethyst will console a mother who feels a sense of abandonment when breastfeeding ends. *Lapis Lazuli*, slipped under the pillow, helps a mother to drop off quickly after nightly feeds. *Sapphire* brings restorative rest and deep sleep. You can also add Amethyst which encourages quality sleep.

Pelvic floor
Strengthening it for life

26 Red Jasper

4 Orange Calcite

24 Fluorite

8 Chinese Green Jade

After giving birth, when the perineum (the area between the vagina and anus, and its underlying muscles) has healed, it is time for pelvic floor exercises together with some form of physiotherapy. Whether you are doing this to avoid stress incontinence or to renew sexual relations with your partner, you can strengthen pelvic muscles by using Geisha, or Ben Wa, balls. These days, similar plastic 'smart' balls in various forms and weights can be bought. Traditionally, however, egg-shaped pieces of *Chinese Green*

Jade were used. The more pointed end makes the stone easy to insert gently and the base of the Jade egg helps you to contract more strongly when the egg is resting on the pelvic floor. The force exerted by the weight of the egg, together with vaginal secretions, enable it to slip out easily when you gently push, as if you were going to urinate. If you cannot find egg-shaped Chinese Green Jade or it is too expensive, you can always use *Red Jasper*, *Fluorite* or *Orange Calcite* crystals instead.

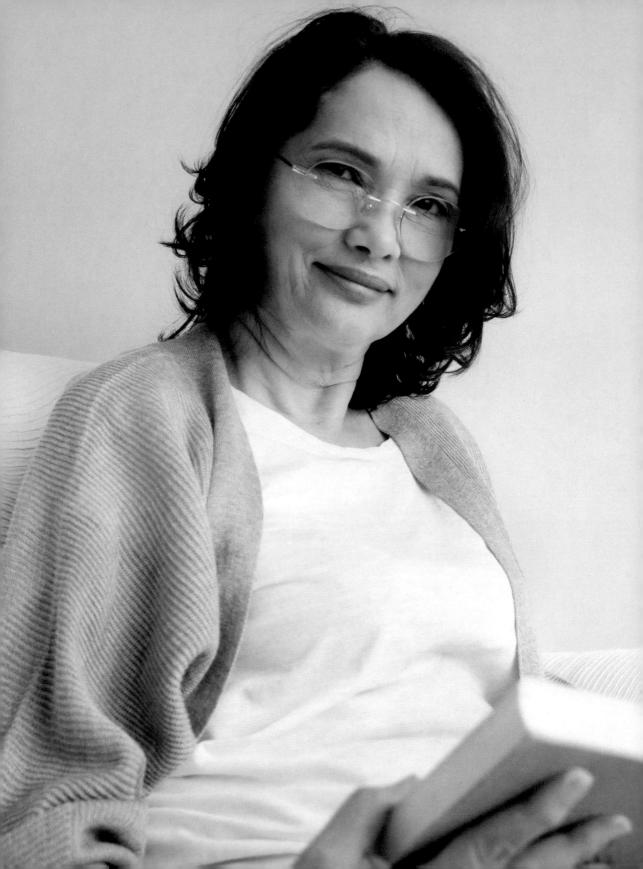

Healing crystals
for later life

An older woman is approaching the autumn of her life, with winter on the horizon. Crystals can be enormously helpful as she faces this new journey, especially when overwhelming, unfamiliar emotions arrive. As her body changes in unexpected ways, the crystals will help her to find stability and fresh energy, which might be different from that of her younger self but just as interesting to experience. Some older women may prefer to use larger, ball-like stones, which are easier to see than little ones that they might lose. Others, who are not physically strong, will opt for small crystals.

Let's take a look at the crystals that can help to navigate through all of this!

The menopause

Everything starts with the menopause, which includes the pre-menopause and post-menopause. Female hormones play havoc with a woman, and for a while she has to juggle with the emotions and many of the problems already encountered in adolescence (see page 60).

Hot flushes
It feels very warm!

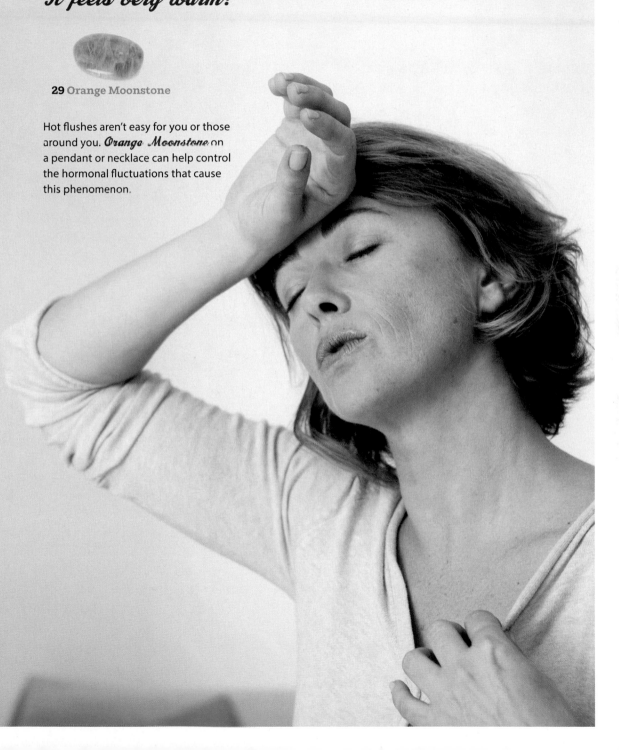

29 Orange Moonstone

Hot flushes aren't easy for you or those around you. *Orange Moonstone* on a pendant or necklace can help control the hormonal fluctuations that cause this phenomenon.

Mood swings & anger
Blame the hormones

   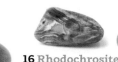

1 Amethyst

5 Chrysoprase

16 Rhodochrosite

29 Orange Moonstone

10 Lilac Lepidolite

3 Blue Chalcedony

Orange Moonstone controls levels of oestrogen and progesterone. *Amethyst* lifts low morale caused by reduced hormone production and helps you to stay in control. To halt mounting anger, try *Chrysoprase*. *Lilac Lepidolite* puts you in a good mood and promotes harmony. *Rhodochrosite* helps settle disputes. *Blue Chalcedony* relieves frustration. Each one can be worn on a necklace, pendant, bracelet or in donut form, or slipped into a pocket. Use them together, too, as you wish.

Sexuality
A strong libido at any age

   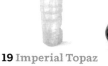

17 Ruby

19 Imperial Topaz

7 Red Garnet

16 Rhodochrosite

14 Tiger's Eye

Menopause-related vaginal dryness can sometimes reduce sexual desire. To rekindle the flame and give yourself a boost, try *Red Garnet*, which will restore your desire and your sexuality. Wear it on a pendant or necklace. *Ruby* stimulates sexual appetite and heightens awareness around the sensitive erogenous zones. *Rhodochrosite* revitalizes sensuality and erotic feelings. *Imperial Topaz* brings tenderness to sexuality. Finally, *Tiger's Eye* makes you daring during sex games. Pelvic exercises with egg-shaped stones also work well and are recommended for sexual comfort and to prevent stress incontinence.

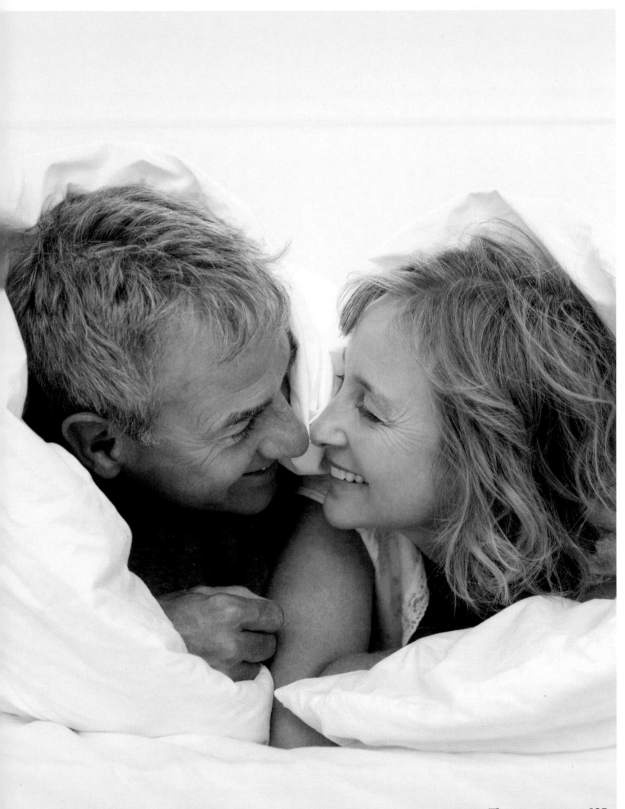

Retirement

Finally some calm arrives with the transition into retirement. But not all women lead this apparently leisurely life. Some take on the role of super grandmother, and happily plunge themselves into a period of intense activity looking after grandchildren. When energy levels start to drop, inactivity can bring contrasting emotions that oscillate between relief and a feeling of uselessness. From a health point of view, it is important to realize that you don't have the same strength you had when you were younger. Time takes its toll. One could say that getting older is the last growth stage. More than ever now, it is essential to have peace of mind and to welcome the good things in life with gratitude.

A hectic life
Staying on top form!

   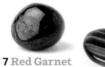 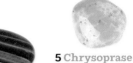

26 Red Jasper   **17** Ruby   **6** Citrine   **7** Red Garnet   **14** Tiger's Eye   **5** Chrysoprase

A helping hand here, looking after grandchildren there, going shopping to help out overstretched offspring … Some grandmothers are very 'useful' and in great demand. Here are some suggestions for sustaining your energy levels and staying fit so that you can maintain your 'super grandmum' image. Try *Red Jasper* to keep up the pace and *Ruby* when you feel worn out (in bracelet, necklace or donut form). *Citrine* will help you to stay happy and smiling when dealing with little terrors. *Red Garnet* will get you through long days. *Tiger's Eye* offers a necessary boost when all you get is 'I don't want to' from the moment they wake up. *Chrysoprase* opens your mind to new experiences with these little adventurers. All of these stones can be worn as you wish.

Adjusting
The world changes so quickly

5 Chrysoprase   **18** Sapphire   **20** Black Tourmaline   **27** Magnetite   **25** Hematite

The older woman has to adapt to the present world with its new, sometimes upsetting rules. *Chrysoprase* encourages you to adjust. Let it dangle from your neck or around your wrist, or slip it into your pocket. *Sapphire* opens your mind to new ideas or experiences. It works well with Chrysoprase. *Black Tourmaline* keeps you rooted in this constantly evolving world and allows you to assimilate the changes. *Magnetite* enables you to refocus when you feel lost. *Hematite* warms and stimulates, making you feel stronger. These crystals can be worn during the day or slipped under the pillow at night.

State of mind
Ups and downs

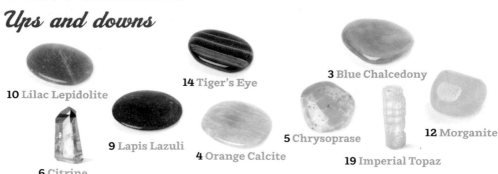

10 Lilac Lepidolite

14 Tiger's Eye

3 Blue Chalcedony

9 Lapis Lazuli

5 Chrysoprase

12 Morganite

4 Orange Calcite

19 Imperial Topaz

6 Citrine

A piece of *Lilac Lepidolite* calms nerves and relieves anxiety. Put it under your pillow at night as it will also encourage drowsiness. During the day, wear it on a pendant or necklace. *Blue Chalcedony* helps you to come out of yourself and seek out other people; above all, avoid turning inwards. Don't forget *Citrine*, which uses all its power to raise morale and bring joy. *Chrysoprase* encourages you to go out and meet new people – perhaps by joining a bridge club or a painting or reading group, or offering educational support. *Tiger's Eye* will give you the incentive to go and find a new physical activity – joining a walking group, attending gentle gym sessions, or Pilates or yoga classes. *Lapis Lazuli* calms troubling thoughts. When it is used with *Imperial Topaz*, it finally brings peace of mind. *Morganite* frees you from emotional or obsessional blockages. Self-confidence returns when you have *Orange Calcite*. These crystals can be worn on a necklace or bracelet, used in donut form or slipped deep into a pocket.

Memory
I've got a mind like a sieve

18 Sapphire

24 Fluorite

20 Black Tourmaline

6 Citrine

15 Rose Quartz

11 Malachite

Here are the top recommendations: *Sapphire* for calming your mind and helping you to express your thoughts; *Fluorite*, preferably blue, which encourages concentration; *Black Tourmaline*, which helps you to focus on the day-to-day. *Citrine* reassures and gives you self-confidence when you've left the shopping list at home. *Rose Quartz* helps to put memory lapses into perspective. And there's nothing better than *Malachite* to combat the fear of forgetting and to avoid stress … which makes you forget everything.

Sleep
Restless nights

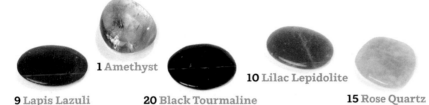

1 Amethyst

10 Lilac Lepidolite

9 Lapis Lazuli

20 Black Tourmaline

15 Rose Quartz

Lapis Lazuli placed on your forehead will encourage drowsiness. An *Amethyst* crystal under your pillow and another on your chest on a necklace or donut pendant will help you sail away into the world of dreams.

Other factors may possibly hinder sleep, such as late nights in front of a computer screen or too much television. These screens emit a blue light that can upset body systems. *Black Tourmaline* reduces the effects of these harmful rays, but if viewing is excessive it can't work miracles. If your nerves are on edge, add *Lilac Lepidolite* placed under your pillow. A good-sized piece of *Rose Quartz* will encourage rest and restorative sleep.

Did you know ...

Physical exercise is essential for older people to maintain cognitive function. Several scientific studies prove it. Taking exercise in the morning is especially recommended. Exercise makes us feel less depressed, less anxious and less angry. The icing on the cake is that it also improves the quality of our sleep. Research from the French INSERM (National Institute of Health and Medical Research) provides plenty of information on this subject. Active women may also live longer, according to a US study published in the *American Journal of Epidemiology* in 2017. The study found that elderly women who were active for less than 40 minutes a day and remained sedentary for more than 10 hours a day had shorter telomeres than their more active peers; telomeres are the tips of DNA strands that protect chromosomes and shorten with age.

Osteoporosis & rheumatism
Careful: brittle bones!

24 Fluorite

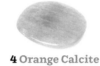

4 Orange Calcite

21 Amber

22 Copper

Multicoloured *Fluorite* encourages the body to use calcium to build strong bones; don't be without it! *Orange Calcite* is another possibility. It brings a sense of peace. Wear it as often as possible, using several Orange Calcite crystals so that you can alternate when one is being cleaned or recharged. *Amber* on a necklace, pendant or bracelet treats joint inflammation and rheumatism. It can be alternated with a piece, or bracelet, of *Copper*. Doctors always recommend regular physical activity. Walking for about 30 minutes a day will strengthen your bone structure. Exercise is also excellent for the memory and for effective brain function.

Mourning
Drowning in tears

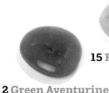

2 Green Aventurine

15 Rose Quartz

12 Morganite

5 Chrysoprase

4 Orange Calcite

16 Rhodochrosite

6 Citrine

Grief is a natural emotion. It allows the body to absorb shock. Normally it does not last too long, but if it persists, you should consult your family doctor or a specialist. *Green Aventurine* opens the heart to accept the loss. *Rose Quartz* reduces the pain. *Morganite* comforts and helps you feel less alone. It also lets you relive happy memories. Lie down for a minute with the crystal on your forehead and imagine there is a tender and happy force travelling to every part of your body. *Rhodochrosite* heals emotional and physical ills. Sadness can be so intense that you feel that your heart has been torn apart. *Chrysoprase* will bring you strength and a sense of renewal. *Orange Calcite* conveys gentleness and hope for the future, while *Citrine* will spread joy and heal the heartache. These crystals can be carried or worn as you wish.

Joy
Staying positive

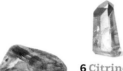
16 Rhodochrosite

6 Citrine

19 Imperial Topaz

4 Orange Calcite

2 Green Aventurine

7 Red Garnet

9 Lapis Lazuli

10 Lilac Lepidolite

It is essential to stay positive and to feel a sense of gratitude and joy within yourself, in your life and in your relationships with other people. A word of thanks to *Rhodochrosite*, the crystal of gratitude; choose a bright pink stone. It fills us with love and encourages us to forgive. *Citrine* brings joy and combats tiredness. Don't forget *Orange Calcite*, which gives a gentle boost, or *Imperial Topaz* which brings serenity. When choosing between these crystals, follow your instinct and pick those that attract you, alternating them according to your mood. Wear them on a necklace or a pendant, in donut form or next to the skin.

Some women have difficulty accepting the loss of the body they had before the menopause. *Green Aventurine* helps them to accept the changes. Wear it on a pendant in the hollow of the neck. Sometimes *Red Garnet* on a necklace or pendant is the best choice. It brings renewed energy when everyday weariness replaces a zest for life. *Lilac Lepidolite* on a necklace, pendant or in donut form puts you in a positive frame of mind. By radiating joy, it provides support at times when you feel depressed. Faced with feelings of 'I can't do this', *Lapis Lazuli* on a necklace, pendant or in donut form helps you to express yourself wisely and without bias. In stressful, deadlock situations when your throat feels tight, this crystal helps to relax it.

Relaxing moments

During a siesta or before you go to sleep, try placing Rhodochrosite – or any other crystal that attracts you – on your forehead, neck, chest, stomach or feet. Following your instincts, you can move the crystal around from place to place and jot down your reactions in your notebook. Practitioners of positive psychology, especially Florence Servan-Schreiber in her book *3 kifs par jour* ('3 daily moments of joy'), (Marabout, 2014) recommends falling asleep while thinking about the good things you've experienced during the day. Feeling grateful can change your mood and give you a sense of well-being. Therefore, the priority is to focus only on good things.

To achieve a different level of consciousness and to experience a sense of peace and serenity, lie down comfortably and place a piece of Rhodochrosite – or Morganite, if preferred – on your heart. These two crystals will transport you to a different dimension. Finally, place a piece of Black Obsidian level with your feet.

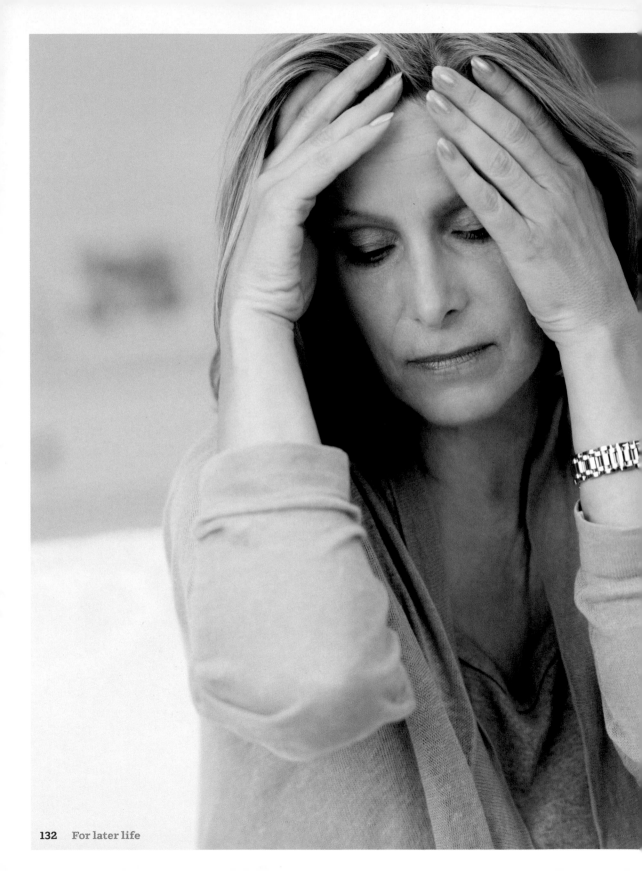

Anxiety
All sorts of fears

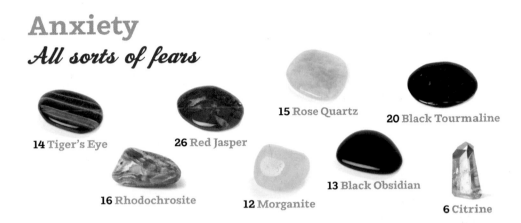

14 Tiger's Eye

26 Red Jasper

15 Rose Quartz

20 Black Tourmaline

16 Rhodochrosite

12 Morganite

13 Black Obsidian

6 Citrine

The school of life never ends. Having to abandon your usual way of doing things and move on and start learning again is not easy. Mastering new skills such as managing crutches or a frame, or finding your way around new places such as a care home is even harder. *Tiger's Eye* helps you to take the plunge and decide to make the change. Carry it in your pocket or wear it on a necklace, bracelet or in donut form. To embrace new things despite a quite understandable fear of change, *Red Jasper* is recommended. This crystal will give you the strength you need. Wearing *Rhodochrosite* will fill you with love that lasts and keeps you positive. To free yourself from recurring or periodically negative emotions, choose *Morganite* and wear it in your bra.

The most effective crystal for deep-seated fears is *Black Obsidian*. Have it with you at night in its raw form or on a necklace or in donut shape. It can be combined with a bracelet or pendant of Rhodochrosite, whose gentleness will fill your heart with tenderness and give you the confidence you lack. You could also hold a ball-shaped piece of *Rose Quartz* and keep it with you for as long as necessary. It is a good idea to combine Black Obsidian with *Black Tourmaline*; using the two crystals together will restore balance where it is needed. Wear them on a pendant, necklace or bracelet.

Fear of death is understandable and reasonable. 'Death is a new sun', said the Swiss-American psychiatrist Elisabeth Kübler-Ross, who was a specialist in support for the dying and a renowned author. Certain crystals, such as *Citrine*, are specifically recommended to encourage a new state of awareness and to relieve this natural and universal fear.

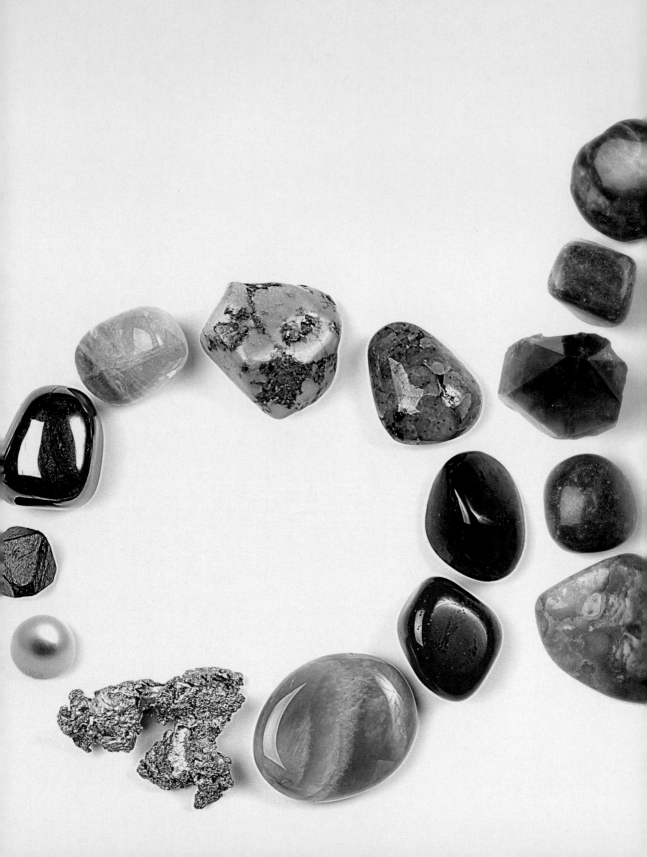

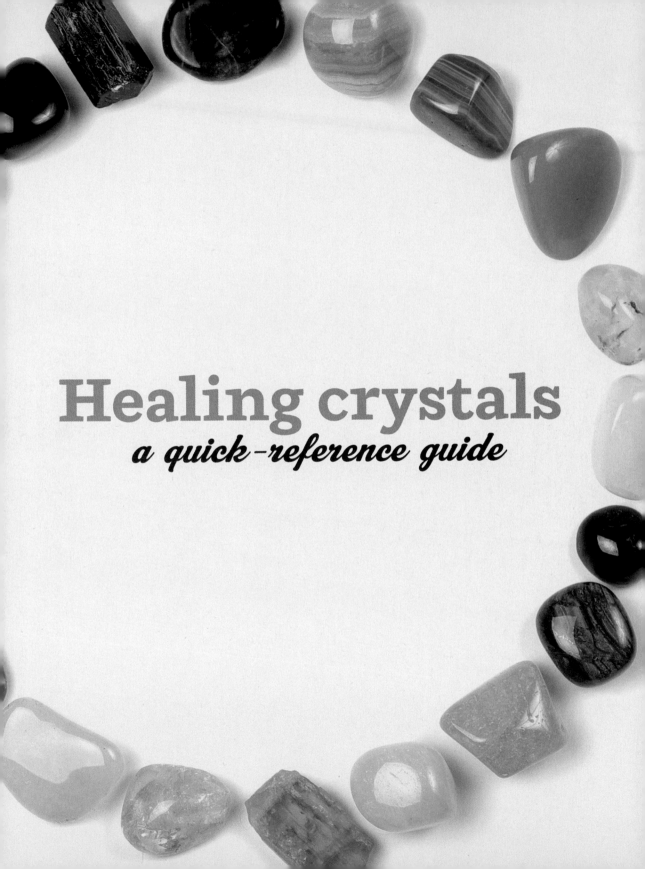

Healing crystals

a quick-reference guide

The 20 essential healing crystals

No.	Name	Description	Family
1	**Amethyst**	• Varying shades of purple from lilac to deep violet • Transparent to translucent • May have milky white lines • Comes in crystal, geode or polished forms	Silicates (when heated turns yellow)
2	**Green Aventurine**	• Green, may be confused with Jade or Emerald	Silicates
3	**Blue Chalcedony**	• Blue with small whitish, parallel lines	Silicates
4	**Orange Calcite**	• Orange, usually polished	Carbonates (various colours forms and crystals)
5	**Chrysoprase**	• Apple green in varying shades from light to dark	Silicates
6	**Citrine**	• Pale yellow, usually heat-treated Amethyst or Smoky Quartz	Silicates
7	**Red Garnet**	• Comes in many colours (green, yellow, pink, brown black) • Can occur as very large crystals	Silicates
8	**Chinese Green Jade or Jadeite or Nephrite**	• Comes in light to dark shades of green and also other colours including purple and white	Silicates
9	**Lapis Lazuli**	• Ultramarine blue with veins of white Calcite or golden pyrite inclusions	Silicates
10	**Lilac Lepidolite**	• Pink to purple	Silicates

Properties	Cleaning	Recharging
Encourages restorative sleep and meditation, relieves headaches, helps you talk to your unborn child, combats fatigue, curbs an excessive appetite, teaches patience	Water + salt Scallop shell	By night, under a rising or full moon Amethyst geode Scallop shell
Encourages acceptance in difficult situations, bereavement, grief, rape, turmoil, mental disquiet, also treats genital-urinary disorders	Water + salt Water + clay Scallop shell	At sunrise Cluster of Quartz/Rock Crystal Scallop shell
Relieves frustration, anxiety, shyness, brings gentleness, encourages speaking out, calms nightmares	Water + salt Water + clay Scallop shell	By night, under a rising or full moon Amethyst geode
Combats gloominess, helps a baby to walk, controls blood pressure, brings confidence and gentle joy, banishes fear	Water + salt Water + clay Scallop shell	At sunrise Cluster of Quartz/Rock Crystal Scallop shell
Encourages change, awareness and contentment, develops femininity, controls over-emotional feelings, comforts sadness, brings emotional security, reduces stress	Water + salt Water + clay Scallop shell	At sunrise Cluster of Quartz/Rock Crystal Scallop shell
Brings joy, good humour, courage and well-being, relieves nausea and lower back pain, reduces conflict, restores emotional balance	Water + salt Water + clay Scallop shell	At sunrise Cluster of Quartz/Rock Crystal Scallop shell
Encourages concentration, action, listening, sexuality, creativity, enthusiasm and courage, boosts blood circulation, combats aching legs, fatigue and timidity, helps during convalescence	Water + salt Water + clay Scallop shell	At sunrise Cluster of Quartz/Rock Crystal Scallop shell
Crystal that brings harmony, wisdom, justice, discernment, patience and determination, soothes anger and guilt, reduces tiredness before childbirth, has a beneficial effect on the kidneys	Water + salt Water + clay Scallop shell	At sunrise Cluster of Quartz/Rock Crystal Scallop shell
Encourages weaning and helps a baby fall asleep, also encourages clear thinking, intuition, effective analysis and communication, brings calm, boosts appetite, soothes away headaches	Water Water + clay Scallop shell	By night, under a rising or full moon Amethyst geode Scallop shell
Boosts morale, has a beneficial effect on emotions and the nervous system, reduces emotional dependence and fears of being abandoned	Water Water + clay Scallop shell	At sunrise Cluster of Quartz/Rock Crystal

continued over →

The 20 essential healing crystals contd.

No.	Name	Description	Family
11	**Malachite**	• Light to dark green	Carbonates
12	**Morganite**	• Pale to lilac pink	Silicates
13	**Black Obsidian**	• Black, sometimes greenish	Silicates and oxides
14	**Tiger's Eye**	• Striped yellow and brown	Silicates
15	**Rose Quartz**	• Opaque or hazy pink in varying shades	Silicates
16	**Rhodochrosite**	• Red to bright pink with lighter layers and white veins	Carbonates
17	**Ruby**	• Opaque red colour • Fine and transparent when used in jewellery	Oxides
18	**Sapphire**	• Brilliant blue, opaque to translucent • Fine gemstone when used in jewellery	Oxides
19	**Imperial Topaz**	• Crystalline, orange to pinkish yellow colour	Silicates
20	**Black Tourmaline**	• Black with one or two pointed ends (either occurring naturally or cut in that way)	Silicates

Properties	Cleaning	Recharging
Reduces anger and resentment, improves judgement, soothes various types of pain, especially kidney pain, relieves minor infections and the effects of traumatic sexual experiences	Water + salt Water + clay Scallop shell	At sunrise Cluster of Quartz/Rock Crystal Scallop shell
Relieves intense sadness, resentment and the effects of traumatic sexual experiences	Water + salt Water + clay Scallop shell	At sunrise Cluster of Quartz/Rock Crystal
Encourages awareness, relieves sadness, guilt and fear, clears emotional blocks, has a beneficial effect on the uterus	Water + salt Water + clay Scallop shell	By night, under a rising or full moon Amethyst geode Scallop shell
Protective crystal, encourages balance and courage, curbs excessive empathy, encourages recuperation, relieves various types of pain	Water + salt Water + clay Scallop shell	At sunrise Cluster of Quartz/Rock Crystal Scallop shell
Brings gentleness, comfort, hope, encourages the mother–daughter relationship, relieves doubt and a baby's fears, encourages optimism	Water + salt Water + clay Scallop shell	At sunrise Cluster of Quartz/Rock Crystal Scallop shell
Controls sensitivity, emotions and anger, encourages communication, calms stress, stimulates libido or treats the effects of traumatic sexual experiences, speeds recovery	Water + salt Water + clay Scallop shell	At sunrise Cluster of Quartz/Rock Crystal Scallop shell
Crystal that encourages vitality, strengthens willpower, drive, courage, boosts blood circulation, speeds recovery	Water + salt Water + clay Scallop shell	At sunrise Cluster of Quartz/Rock Crystal Scallop shell
Calms nerves, oversensitivity and stress, encourages communication, tranquillity and meditation	Water + salt Water + clay Scallop shell	At sunrise Cluster of Quartz/Rock Crystal Scallop shell
Calms nerves and oversensitivity, encourages communication, strengthens, encourages optimism, treats the endocrine glands, the liver, the gall-bladder, and relieves the effects of traumatic sexual experiences	Water + salt Water + clay Scallop shell	At sunrise Cluster of Quartz/Rock Crystal Scallop shell
Reassures, encourages stability, grounding, a positive frame of mind and awareness, protects against radiation	Water + salt Water + clay Scallop shell	At sunrise Cluster of Quartz/Rock Crystal Scallop shell

The 10 'bonus' crystals

No.	Name	Description	Family
21	**Amber**	• Yellow with bubbles, fractures and sometimes suspended fossilized insect and plant parts	Organic compound Fossilized conifer resin
22	**Copper**	• Golden yellow	Metals
23	**Emerald**	• Green • Sparkling green when used in jewellery	Silicates
24	**Fluorite**	• Colourless, green, pink, purple, blue	Fluorines
25	**Hematite**	• Greyish brown or brownish red, iridescent	Oxides
26	**Red Jasper**	• Red, but also many other colours	Silicates
27	**Magnetite**	• Greyish brown	Oxides
28	**Freshwater Pearl**	• Pinkish to orange white • As a gem, greyish white in varying shades	Carbonates
29	**Orange Moonstone**	• Greyish to orange milky white	Silicates
30	**Turquoise**	• Bright blue to green, veined with black	Phosphates

Properties	Cleaning	Recharging
Relieves toothache, breast pain and stomach pains, treats ulcers, chapped skin and acne, boosts vitality	Water + salt Water + clay Scallop shell	At sunrise Cluster of Quartz/Rock Crystal
Relieves pain and inflammation, controls greasy hair, calms the mind, helps to eliminate toxins, speeds recovery	Laid on clay Scallop shell	At sunrise Cluster of Quartz/Rock Crystal Scallop shell
Detoxifies, controls greasy hair, relieves acne, soothes tired eyes, reduces anger, encourages determination and harmony	Water + salt Water + clay Scallop shell	At sunrise Cluster of Quartz/Rock Crystal Scallop shell
Encourages concentration, open-mindedness, strengthens tendons, teeth and bones	Water + salt Water + clay Scallop shell	At sunrise Cluster of Quartz/Rock Crystal
Speeds recovery, encourages iron absorption, stimulates	Laid on clay Scallop shell	At sunrise Cluster of Quartz/Rock Crystal
Helps turn ideas into reality, encourages self-confidence, drive and vitality, treats circulation problems, stress, constipation and cramp	Water + salt Water + clay Scallop shell	By night, under a rising or full moon Amethyst geode
Encourages you to refocus, achieve and shine, relieves cramp, treats leg pain	Laid on clay Scallop shell	By night, under a rising or full moon Amethyst geode
Develops a woman's attractiveness, reduces water retention and relieves stomach pains	Water Scallop shell	At sunrise Cluster of Quartz/Rock Crystal
Useful during pregnancy, childbirth and breastfeeding, beneficial effect on hormones	Water + salt Water + clay Scallop shell	By night, under a rising or full moon Amethyst geode
Protective crystal, encourages communication, personal development and creativity	Water + clay Scallop shell	At sunrise Cluster of Quartz/Rock Crystal Scallop shell

Index

Acknowledgements

We would like to thank Leduc.s ´Editions for their faith in us. We would also like to offer special thanks to M. Éclancher, manager of Minerals of Brazil, located in the 8th arrondissement of Paris. Both of us worked in that store, selling and advising customers about crystals, and it is where we had the good fortune to meet each other. The path that we still pursue together gives us the opportunity to offer you the knowledge that we have gained.

Catherine and Nathaëlh

Picture credits

Eddison Books Limited
Creative Consultant **Nick Eddison**
Managing Editor **Tessa Monina**
Translation, design and editorial **3redcars.co.uk**
Proofreader **Nikky Twyman**
Indexer **Marie Lorimer**
Production **Sarah Rooney & Cara Clapham**